There's something
BEHIND THAT
Smile

There's Something Behind That Smile
Copyright@2017 by Dorothy Wyrick

All rights reserved. No part of this publication may be reproduced or transmitted in any form or by any means, electronic or mechanical, including photocopying, recording or by any information storage and retrieval system, without permission in writing from the publisher.

Unless, otherwise indicated, Scripture quotations are from the translations of the New King James Holy Bible
& New King James Version (Spirit Filled Life Bible for Students)

Wyrick, Dorothy
There's Something Behind that Smile

1.Liver 2. Organs 3. Transplant 4. Faith 5. Recovery 6. Memoir 7. African American Health

ISBN-13: 978-1541240476
ISBN-10: 1541240472

First Edition

10 9 8 7 6 5 4 3 2

Printed in United States of America

DEDICATION

I dedicate this book to everyone who has been a part of my life, and to those who have touched my heart in a tremendous way. To all my dearest friends, family, coworkers at the Federal Center, and church family. To my spiritual father Bishop Hugh D. Smith, Jr. (founder of Emmanuel Covenant Church International in Battle Creek, Michigan), his beautiful wife Letha, their three gorgeous daughters, and two grandsons–The Tiny Princes.

Much love to Senior Pastor Frederick J. Sweet, his lovely wife, Co-Pastor Shannon Sweet, and their two precious daughters.

To my handsome father, Willie Mann Jr., my lovely mother, Ola B. Mann, and to my loveable stepmother Ethel Mann. Thank you all for being there when I needed you the most. And to my fine, loving husband who inspired me to pursue the impossible–my dream. I will always love you. Thank you all for being a witness to my healing, which is shared in the pages of this book. I love you all dearly, in Jesus' name.

To my readers:
It's time to get plugged in and connected to our Heavenly Father so we can have a relationship with Him. Learn to love yourself, recognize that we are unique and peculiar people. No one is like you! Enjoy the blessing of life with the people who treasure you every day.

For the moment, can we forgive and move on? Have you ever wondered why the most unhappy people are the ones who lack something to make them happy? I call them lost, because they know not Jesus.

Try not to get caught up in the frustrating circumstances of today and let them get you down. Appreciate living! Trials and storms will come. Trust in God, have faith, and believe that trouble only lasts for a season. "Do not let your hearts be troubled" (John 14:1). Live for the moment–now! Let go and let God do the rest.

D.W.

In the beginning was the Word, and the Word was with God, and the Word was God.

John 1:1

TABLE OF CONTENTS

Introduction

Poem- *I Am*- 11

Chapter One – *Who Am I?*- 13

Chapter Two - *What's Going On?*- 21

Chapter Three - *Here for a Purpose*- 31

Chapter Four - *In the Meantime*- 49

Chapter Five - *The Wait*- 61

Chapter Six - *Who Can Find a Virtuous Woman?*- 71

Chapter Seven – *Story of Job*- 85

Chapter Eight - *You got to put a ring on it!*- 91

Chapter Nine - *The Operation*- 107

Chapter Ten – *There's No Place Like Home*- 125

Chapter Eleven - *The Wedding*- 133

Poem: Smile- 144

Afterword- 145

The Virtuous Woman I Am- 146

A Love Letter Dedication- 149

History & Notes: Primary Biliary Cirrhosis (PBC)- 155

Glossary- 163

The Future- 172

In Memory- 173

Conclusion & Acknowledgements- 176

About the Author- 177

I shall not die, but live, and declare the works of the Lord.

Psalm 118:17

INTRODUCTION

You never know when a trial or tribulation may come your way. I had always heard people in the church say, "You need to prepare for an unexpected roller coaster ride called, A Test of Faith." They were saying that a crisis will come, so be prepared. I knew this ride all too well.

I had already experienced heartache in my life through the loss of my beloved grandmothers. I was left to raise a child as a single mother and thought I would never find true love. I allowed myself to be taken for granted. However, all of that paled in comparison to what was to come.

For years, I had unexplained itching all over my body that could only be soothed by the sharp objects I used to relieve the chronic irritation. It was so bad that I had thoughts of suicide. I just wanted the itching to stop. I lost so much weight that some people thought I had been using drugs. My physical body was weak, vulnerable and confused. I felt helpless when the doctors in my hometown of Battle Creek, Michigan had no idea what was going on.

The complications from this unknown illness led me to retire early from my job at the Battle Creek Federal Center where I had worked as a federal civilian for more than twenty-six years. My mind would say, "Throw in the towel and quit, but my heart said, That's not what God wants."

In 2000, I was admitted into Battle Creek Health System where I was diagnosis with a rare liver disease that had slowly destroyed my bile ducts. The bile ducts carry bile from the liver to the small intestine to help digest fat. The only thing that could save me was a liver transplant. Never realizing I would have such a test of faith, I did as the Saints at church had suggested for years, to "Get Ready", as the test of storms will come. I prepared for the roller coaster ride and put all my faith in my heavenly Father whom I had known since the age of five.

The ride was scary at times, but I put my trust in the Lord. I went through treatments and was placed on the list for a liver transplant. As an African American, organ donation was not something discussed. The thought of giving away organs that we may one day need our self was unthinkable. Even donating organs after our death was rarely considered.

As I learned more about my failing liver, I realized that there may have been others in my family who suffered from this as well. But, they did not know it and died without ever receiving treatment. I am one of the few survivors of a liver transplant made possible by a donation from someone who was not an immediate family member.

I want the world to know my story. I want to help educate African Americans about this illness and the trial of an organ transplant. I was heavenly blessed to have a second chance at life. I am healed, healthy, a blessing to be a blessing to others, a miracle from heaven and a woman after God's own heart.

I believe in my heart that God created people to be tested and to go through tribulations so they can make history. I cannot reserve this testimony for the people who know me. It is time to tell my story to the world. It is a story of the goodness and healing Jesus has done for me. I recognize that He is the Way, the Truth, and the Light. It feels so good to be happy in Christ.

I'm writing about my life experience as a true, living, walking testimony, while reflecting on basic biblical references that have sustained me on this path. I have learned that life is not a Cinderella story to live happily ever after. Of course, there will be trials. You will get through them with prayer, education in organ transplantation, and a desire to live. Through the pages of this book, I pray my spiritual experiences will help you grow deeper in hope, faith and in the healing power of God.

This is my story based on my testimony of truth and long suffering. Before you begin to read, cuddled up in a soft warm blanket and relax with a hot cup of tea. Clear your thoughts of all your troubles. Open your *heart* and focus on our *Heavenly Father* whom created us. Here in the pages to come, I share with you all the pain I endured.

I also share of the joy I found when I took my journey through organ transplantation with *prayer, hope, patience, faith, belief, forgiveness, laughter, healing, love* and standing on God's Word to deliver me from sickness to health.

Keep your heart with all diligence, for out of it springs the issue of life.

Proverbs 4:23

Keep yourselves in the love of God, looking for the mercy of our Lord Jesus Christ unto eternal life.

Jude 1:21

I AM

I am a Godly woman.
I am truth. I am honest.
I am strong. I am to be successful.
I am rich in Jesus' name, I am healed, I am highly favored.
I am the head and not the tail; I am brilliant, I am happy. I am blessed.

I am healthy. I am wisdom.
I am a writer.
I am money, I am wealth, I am future, I am destiny.
I am joyful, I am lovable.
I am sunshine, light and lovely.
I am funny, I am smiles, I am confident.
I am anointed and of good character.
I am Queen, I am beautiful inside and out. I am kind.
I am married and loving it!

I am a child of God, a miracle, a Christian.
I am the oldest child and a family of hope. I have been tested.
I am a stable, caring, positive inspiration who people love.
I am pleasant, mature and a light of the world.

I am special and unique, wearing the blessing created from God to represent Him – I am the gift of healing and I am thankful every day of my life to be alive!

I have stepped out on faith to tell the world about the love of Jesus Christ.

I am not a quitter but a winner; never looking back I will continue my course. I am getting out of debt.
I am an author!

Chapter 1

WHO AM I?

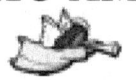

Someone once told me that I would be nothing in life. I was criticized for having a child out of wedlock and was told I would never be loved as Christ loves me. I was told I would never get married and that I was "fake" because I smiled so much. Even in my sickness with liver disease someone said that I would not be healed. Others said that I was too old to dream. I am a woman who can truly shout the lyrics of Chaka Khan's, "I'm Every Woman!" More importantly, "I'm a Godly Woman that loves to Praise the Lord!"

Why do I smile? Sorry, Pastor Joel Osteen, I think I have you beat when it comes to showing my pearly whites. Being able to smile is a gift from God who created me to be an image of Him in the eyes of the world...smile and all. When I was younger, I smiled to be seen as a good little girl. As I became a teenager, I smiled to have friends and get some attention from boys (who took that smile the wrong way). In my adult years, I smiled to keep the peace and to get along with everyone. But throughout my life, situations were upon me that would have led others to wonder if they could ever, be real, with a genuine smile from inside out. Now, I know why I smile.

My spiritual foundation began in the church when I was a child. Everyone on my father's side of the family was a part of the church. My grandfather, Willie Mann Sr., was a pastor who passed the baton to my uncles, Elder Joseph and Pastor David Mann. My first cousin Edmon Mann and his wife Mary are pastors in Albion, MI. Dr. Janice Holmes-Mann and her husband Bennie Holmes are pastors in Detroit, MI. My grandmothers Lizzie Mann and Arzola Edwards were truly virtuous women. Through their examples of walking in faith, I knew deep down in my soul and heart that there was nothing too big or too small for God.

When I was younger, I thought it would be cool to smoke cigarettes like the famous actress Betty Davis. When I inhaled, I choked. That was the end of my smoking. When I was 18 years old, our high school senior class took a trip to Mexico. In America, we were not the legal drinking age, but we took it upon ourselves to sample the infamous Tequila drink with the worm. When I tried it, I got so sick I thought I was going to die.

While in the hotel room (while everyone else was enjoying the sites) my friend Kristena Drain kept a cool towel on my forehead in her pretend nurse role. Her response to me, "What were you thinking about?" I said, "I wasn't thinking at all." She was a true friend who stayed right there by my side until I was able to get back on my feet. At the same time, my desire to "fit in" as a drinker was over.

The test of faith would be needed more than ever one morning in 2000. It was on this particular day I went to get out of bed as usual. Only this time as my feet hit the floor, I fell. My daughter was living on her own and raising her children. I worked at the Federal Center in Battle Creek and to this point enjoyed the solitude of living alone and single. After all, I made sure to live a healthy lifestyle. I was not a health fanatic but I made the right choices based on traumatic circumstances that influenced my decisions.

As an adult I made sure my lifestyle was to exercise three or four days a week at the local YMCA and keep my "high" limited to spiritual walks with Jesus. "Set your affection on things above and not things in the earth" (Colossians 3:2). With these practices, I just knew I would be in excellent shape forever. But as my grandmother would say, "Just keep on living."

"Do you need to see a priest?" the nurse asked.

If that is what I needed, I was to request it now. There was no guarantees once surgery began- no matter how routine – that I will come out alive. I knew that.

"No, I have the Most High God right here by my side, living inside of me. Thanks anyway," I said smiling as usual.

I had been praying for years–even before I knew my diagnosis–for God to ease the pain that riddled my body. After I had been accepted on the liver transplant list I prayed for months to let it come in a timely fashion. I have been praying for hours as my father drove and stepmother, Ethel, rode with us within the three hours (as she did so often through the years) to Northwestern Memorial Hospital in Chicago, to allow this surgery to be a success. Today, I would receive my liver transplant and it was faith that had brought me along this seven-year journey.

Despite my quest for healthy living, "life" happened. I had acquired a rare chronic liver disease that destroyed by bile ducts, making it impossible for my liver to function properly. Life on my job had been a struggle for years. Some family members were in denial when I needed them the most, especially, when I had no clue why I had gone from 160 pounds to 90 pounds overnight. No, I didn't need a priest.

The nurse returned with a small pill to help relax my stomach while the IV was in my arm. As I lay on the bed, prepped for surgery, my father and Ethel held my hand and prayed. Whatever, I had been given began to take affect and I was slowly slipping into a deep sleep. They both looked at me with a big smile and kissed me. I couldn't talk, but my smile was letting them know how much I appreciated and loved them for their care throughout this journey. My dad never missed a beat when it came to driving me to Chicago for a follow-up visits.

When I was told I could only be saved through a liver transplant, he did not know how much longer he would have his daughter and did everything possible to ease my pain. He had done all he could. Dad soon stepped back. Now, it was God's turn to step in and show the world what He could do through me and through this transplant.

I felt the bed being pushed away from Daddy and Ethel. I wished they could come with me. As my eyes got heavier, I also felt myself being wheeled down the hall to the surgery room. I quietly murmured to myself, "Lord, forgive me of all my sins. And if I have done anything that wasn't pleasing to you, please, please forgive me, in Jesus' name."

And the prayer of faith shall save the sick, and the Lord shall raise him up: and if he have committed sins, they shall be forgiven him.
James 5:15

Once I entered the operating room, I saw big bright light and people with white masks standing around the table looking at me. My vision was slowly fading away. I tried to smile and say "Hello" as a simple courtesy upon entering a room (that is what I had been taught). However, I could not utter a word. My eyelids grew too heavy to hold open as I began to think about my life, and the unfinished purpose here on earth.

What is God's plan for my life?

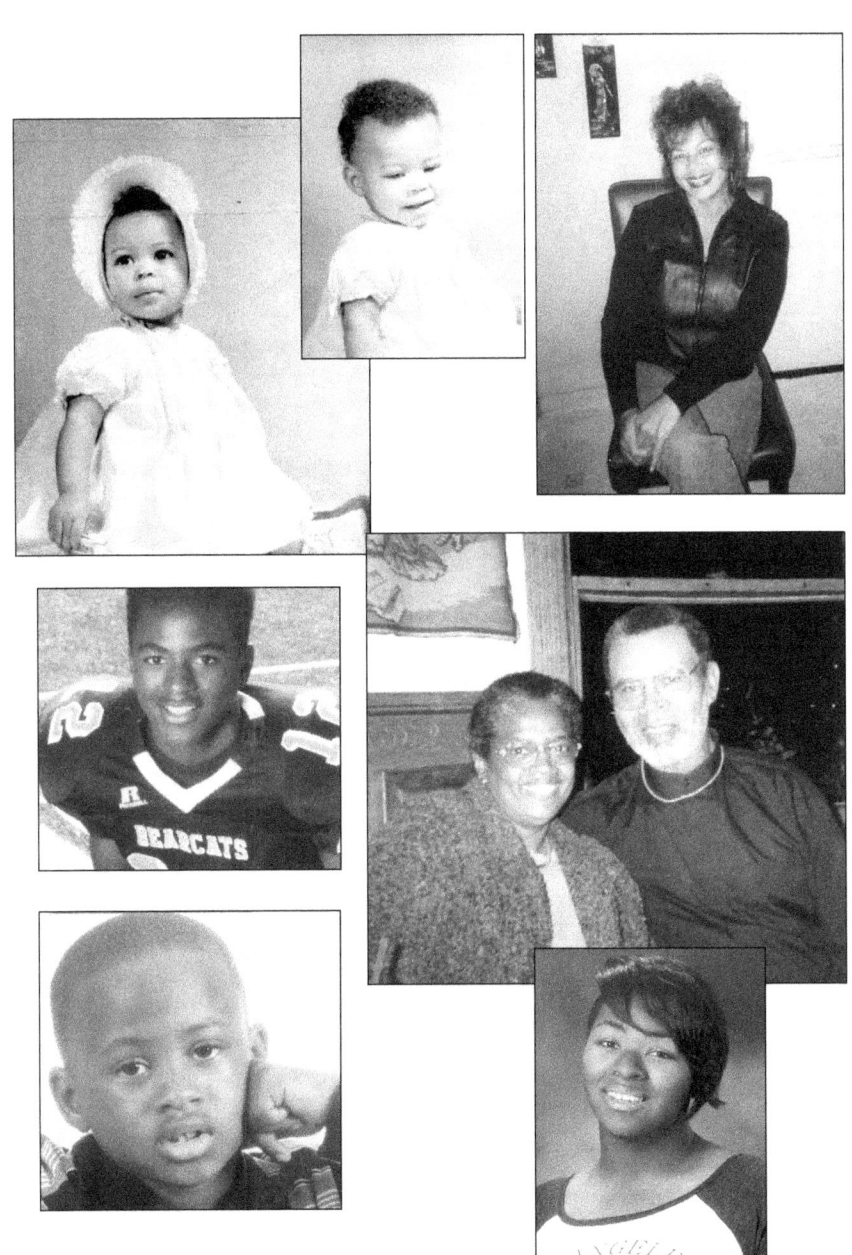

Clockwise: My baby pictures with my signature smile; me before my diagnosis; my father Willie Mann Jr. and his wife, Ethel; my grandchildren: Jasmine Warren, Joshua Mann, and Juan Warren II.

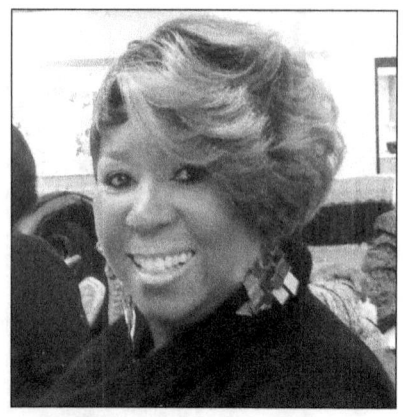
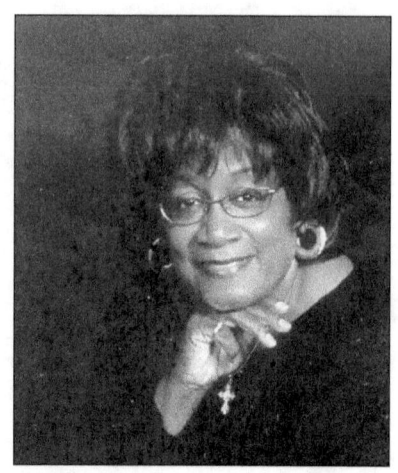
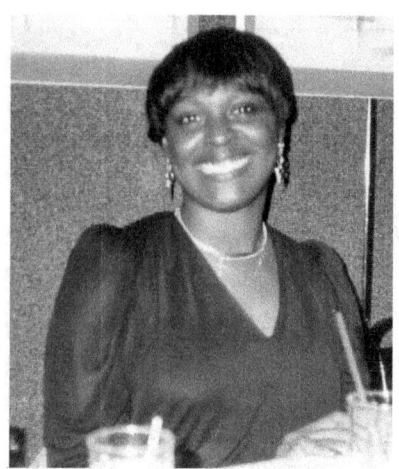
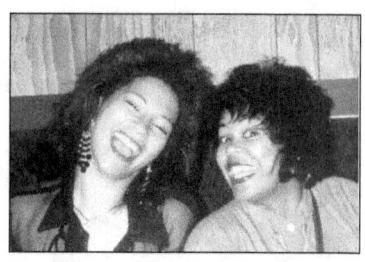
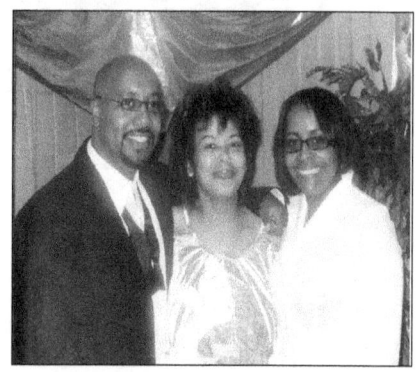
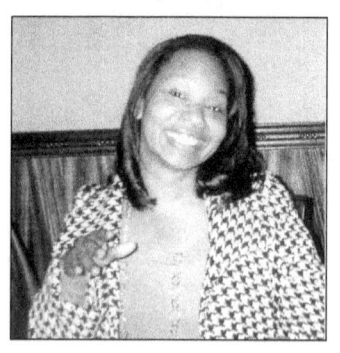

Clockwise: My best friends Jeanette "Nippy" Broadway, Michelle Franklin and I, my pastor, Bishop Hugh Smith Jr. and his wife, First Lady Letha Smith (me in the center), Katie Barnes, Esther Harden; and my cousin Dr. Janice Holmes.

*Let everything that hath breath praise the Lord.
Praise ye the Lord.*

Psalm 150:6

Chapter 2

WHAT'S GOING ON?

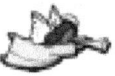

I was three months old when *The Wizard of Oz* debuted on television in November of 1956. My parents, Ola Edwards and Willie Mann Jr., and my father's brother Joseph, had grown up seeing the movie in theater. Once I was born, Uncle Joseph insisted I be named Dorothy (so the story goes).

As their firstborn child, they coddled over their little fair-skinned daughter whose face was sprinkled with a few brown freckles. My nose was no bigger than a pop cap and I had a few curls in the front of my head to take the attention off the back of my head, which was completely bald. My grandmother Arzola, informed me that I was an ugly duckling. She was glad that I had "grew-up into a lovely swan with a beautiful personality."

I grew up relatively healthy, physically that is. I fell in love with my high school sweetheart who left me to raise our daughter alone as a single parent. Despite the bumps and bruises of relationships I was pretty content and held a great job at the Federal Center in my hometown of Battle Creek.

In 2001, my whole life would take a new meaning. That year, my daughter Nicole had her third child, Joshua. Soon after, I was ask to perform duties as a grandmother and watched her children while she worked. For some reason, when I went to hold him I began to itch uncontrollably. I was hoping I was not allergic to my grandchild. Whatever the reason, it was impossible for me to care for him.

In the last few months, it seems like living with this itching turn my life upside down. As days and nights were passing, my condition was not getting any better, but it was not getting worse, either. God's word is not to worry or doubt, but trust in Him.

*Trust in the Lord with all thine heart; and lean not unto thine own
understanding. In all your ways acknowledge him
and he will direct your path.*
Proverb 3:5

Around this same time, I noticed that I was losing weight. My usual weight of about 175 pounds had decreased to 150 pounds without dieting. I took this weight loss as a chance to wear smaller, cute stylish outfits that I have admired in stores for years. It was fun spending and buying new petite clothes! At the same time, I had a loss of energy that I just attributed to overextending myself.

I never complained about it but continue to keep smiling. Regardless, how unpleasant my situation was. I smiled as I worked my full-time job, as I prepared cakes for church events or special occasions. I continued with my every day routine, forty hours of work, writing poetry, exercising at the YMCA and baby sitting while my daughter worked the night shift as a single parent.

One day while at work, I had an uncontrollable itch. I had been feeling that same itch for a few weeks. Maybe it was something in the air at the office.

"Is anyone itching beside me?" I asked my coworkers who were sitting at their desks. Everyone laughed, so I did too, and just dropped the subject. I did not want anyone to think I was going crazy.

I am NOT crazy. I have never had experience anything like this in my whole life! I continued to sit there and try to perform my duties while I itched and scratched as little as possible. Then, one night while giving my grandson a bottle, my hands and feet started itching. I even noticed how my skin would easily bruise with the slightest pressure of a scratch.

When I fell out of bed one morning, I took it as exhaustion and shrugged it aside. I was nauseous and fatigue. I thought, maybe I was just tired. My friends began to point out my physical changes. Others began to take notice – or at least say something to me about my symptoms as opposed to not talking about me behind my back. I can say, "The only true friends I do have are real friends with a heart."

My friend and coworker, Jeanette "Nippy" Broadway, was the first to notice that my skin was turning a lighter shade. She said that she knew of another person whose skin had got lighter when it has something to do with their liver. Somehow, that didn't make sense to me, so I shrugged it off.

Another friend, Marilyn Morris echoed Nippy's concerns. "Is there something going on with your liver?" she asked. And like Nippy, she suggested that I go to see a doctor and have it checked out. I still didn't take it seriously. Since I hadn't experienced any type of skin discoloration before. There is no need to rush, just because everyone requested it.

One day my friend, Esther Harden and I stop by my mother's house on our way to the Federal Center picnic. My mother kept staring at my weight and eyes. Then, like my mother, they noticed my yellowing eyes and that I didn't have as much pep as usual. She looked worried and confused. As I quickly walked toward the door to leave, I smiled and kissed her. My friends Esther and Katie Barnes notice my sudden weight loss too. Esther was so funny.

She said to Katie and me, "What is Dot doing?"

Esther replied, "I am going to start following her around to see how she is losing weight so fast." We all laughed.

Through all of their observations, I was still smiling. My natural ability to be happy spiritually is a gift from God. I have always tried to find the positive in everything. Without ever reading popular, self-help books I knew that attitude plays an important role in thoughts and actions.

My stubborn pride was more than my friends could take. They insist I go to the doctor. After months of major discomfort, I just could not ignore their request any longer. Maybe it will be something simple that I should have taken care from the beginning. Whatever it was, it would be a simple fix, I thought. I promised myself to make an appointment, later.

As the weeks went on, I couldn't rest. At some point, I would itch so badly that I wanted to knock on my neighbor's door to ask them to drive me to the hospital. But my pride got in the way. One night, pride had to be set aside as I headed towards the Mabry's house for help. As I open the car door to get out and knock, I immediately shut it. I could not take another step. I had to drive myself to the hospital, now!

In haste and possible delirium, I almost struck a tree. My strength was gone but God helped me quickly to avoid any accidents. I prayed that I would make it to the emergency room. Once I arrived, I tried my best to explain what had been happening over the past months. I was checked into a room and hooked to an IV with medication that would sooth my itching. Once the itching was under control, I was discharged. I thought!

Throughout the rest of the night and next day, the itching started again. I realized I needed to see a doctor who could have more time to analyze me than those in the emergency room. My friend, Michelle Franklin, referred me to her doctor and scheduled the appointment. On the day of the appointment, she and Esther took off work to support me.

After the nurse drew blood, the doctor returned with the test results. As the doctor read the verdict, I sat there with a smile and believed in God's word to trust in Him. She looked at the lab work and then at me.

"You have Primary Biliary Cirrhosis of the liver," she read.

I guess I didn't understand. My usual easy smile began to quiver. The doctor described my symptoms, but at the same time, she was amazed that I was still walking around at all after having such chronic symptoms without any treatment.

"Your liver enzymes are wacky and out of control," she said explaining the seriousness of the diagnosis. "By this time, you should have been dead."

"What are you talking about?" I said confused. She couldn't believe how in the world I was still walking around.

She told me that my liver was not functioning properly; it is failing. I was in shock but still optimistic. I assumed that because I was still alive it was something medication could cure. Wrong!

I looked at Michelle and Esther as the doctor said that simple medication was not an option. She explained that, "Primary Biliary Cirrhosis (PBC) is, a rare chronic liver disease that slowly destroys the bile ducts. Liver inflammation over a period of years causes scarring, which leads to cirrhosis. The cause of PBC is unknown and because of the varying symptoms, diagnosis can sometimes be overlooked. It is considered as autoimmue disease, in which the body turns against its own cells.

She told me that women are affected ten times more than men, and that PBC, an autoimmune disease, is usually diagnosed in patients between the ages of 30 to 60. While I was losing weight, the doctor said that many with PBC usually look extremely healthy and may even be ten to thirty pounds overweight. She said that usually, there is a slight bronze pigmentation of the skin that gives an appearance of a tan. My skin was having the opposite effect; it was getting lighter.

The outward appearance may not tell the whole story of what is going on inside the body, but it does give you important clues. My friends and I were all educated in the office that day. We learned is often associated with one or more autoimmune diseases such as Rheumatoid Arthritis Syndrome, Raynaud's, Lupus, or Scleroderma.

What I learned that day:

Upon diagnosis, patients are advised to avoid alcohol. There can be dark urine, gray, yellow or light-colored stools; nausea, vomiting and/or loss of appetite; vomiting of blood, bloody or black stools. Intestinal bleeding can occur when disease obstruct blood flow through the liver.

The bleeding may result in blood or bloody stools and abdominal swelling. Liver disease may cause ascites, an accumulation of abdominal cavity, prolonged, generalized itching, and unusual changes in weight. Sleep disturbances, mental confusion, and coma are present in severe liver disease as a result from an accumulation of toxic substances in the body. This may lead to fatigue or loss of stamina, and absence of periods in women and a lack of sexual desire.

The liver is the largest organ in the body. It is found high in the right upper abdomen behind the ribs and is a more complex organ than I ever imagined. Its many functions include:

- Stores energy in the form of sugar (glucose),

- Stores vitamins, iron and other minerals,

- Makes proteins, including blood-clotting factors to keep the body healthy and help grow,

- Processes worn-out red blood cells; making bile which is needed for food digestion,

- Metabolizes or break down many medication and alcohol, and kill germs that enter the body through the intestine.

- The live cells excrete bile into tiny tubes within the liver called bile ducts. These tubes come together like the tiny veins on a leaf. They drain the bile into the common bile duct, a large single tube leading into the intestine. There the bile aids digestion and gives stool its brown color. As you can see, the liver is a very important organ.

What is Primary Biliary Cirrhosis (PBC)?

Primary Biliary Cirrhosis is a disease of the bile duct inside the liver. It progresses slowly and patients may lead active, productive lives for many years. In PBC, the bile ducts in the liver become inflamed. The inflammation is chronic (constant over a long period of time), and causes scaring that eventually blocks and destroys the bile ducts.

This condition interferes with the proper drainage of bile, so the bile backs up into the liver and into the bloodstream causing various symptoms. Eventually the liver itself becomes badly damaged and scarred. This is known as cirrhosis.

The exact cause of PBC is unknown. Scientists believe there could be more than one contributing factor. While it does not have the traits of an inherited disease, it does appear more often in some families. People with PBC sometimes have a history of allergies or autoimmune disturbances (that is when the body's immune system recognizes a part of the body as foreign and injures or goes to war against it).

Many patients have no symptoms in the early stages of the disease. The only finding may be abnormal blood laboratory results. For example, a high level of the liver enzyme called alkaline phosphates may be formed in the blood. Itching and fatigue are common symptoms later in the disease. Itching is caused by bile entering the bloodstreams.

As PBC progresses other symptoms occur. There may be jaundice (yellowing of skin and eyes from excess bile in the blood), cholesterol deposits in the skin, fluid accumulation and darkening of the skin. Other immune-related problems may also be present. Arthritis and thyroid problems may be present, and osteoporosis can develop in later stages. The bones become soft and fragile, leading to increased risk of fractures. The development of cirrhosis is the end result of PBC.

A PBC diagnosis is based on several pieces of information. Itching and fatigue alert the physician that bile ducts may be damaged. As previously mentioned, high levels of certain liver enzymes in the blood are important clues. Some people don't understand that the liver plays a key role in converting food into essential chemicals that leave the stomach and pass through the liver before reaching the body. The liver is thus strategically placed to process nutrients and drugs into the digestive tract in forms that are easier for the rest of the body to use. In essence it is the body's refinery.

Your liver plays a principal role in removing from the blood digestive internally – produced toxic substances. The liver converts them to substances that are eliminated from the body.

Your liver helps you by:
- Producing quick energy when it is needed,
- Manufacturing new body proteins,
- Preventing shortages in body fuel by storing certain vitamins & minerals,
- Regulating transport of fat stores,
- Regulating blood clotting,
- Aiding in the digestive process by producing bile,
- Controlling the production and excretion of cholesterol,
- Neutralizing and destroying poisonous substances,
- Metabolizing alcohol,
- Monitoring and maintain the proper level of many chemicals and drugs,
- Cleansing the blood and discharging waste products into the bile,
- Maintaining hormone balance,
- Serving as the main organ of blood formation before birth,
- Helping the body resist infection by producing immune factors and regenerating its own damaged tissue and storing iron.

For God, who commanded the light to shine in our hearts, to give the light of the knowledge of the glory of God in the face of Jesus Christ.

II Corinthians 4:6

Chapter 3

HERE FOR A PURPOSE

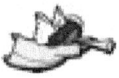

After what seemed like a college science lecture on the liver, the doctor said that I was at a stage where there was only one option – a liver transplant. The good news was that 90% of those who receive a liver transplant are still alive more than a year after the transplant. The bad news was that the number of those waiting for a liver transplant far outweighs the number of organs donated.

But several new developments in transplantation may make it possible for more people to receive the organs they desperately need. These developments include the donation of liver segments from living relatives, splitting one donated liver between two recipients, new organ allocation policies and, especially, new approaches to liver transplants for people with Hepatitis C.

Blocked or inflamed bile ducts are a fluid that aids in the digestion of fats. It's produced in your liver and travels to your gallbladder and small intestine (duodenum) through thin tubes called bile ducts. Diseases such as PBC can cause the ducts to become inflamed, scarred or blocked. This forces bile back into the liver, where it damages tissue and eventually may lead to cirrhosis.

Complications from surgery on the liver, bile ducts or gallbladder (secondary biliary cirrhosis) also can lead to bile ducts being blocked. Babies sometimes develop cirrhosis as a result of biliary atresia–a condition in which the bile ducts are closed or missing at birth.

My reaction from the medical report was, "Oh my God, this is unbelievable! WOW, it's a lot to swallow in one day, 2 hours and 15 seconds, then exhale. Will somebody pinch me – tell me it's only a dream!"

I looked at my friends. We didn't want to believe what we had just heard.

"I don't believe it!" Once we were back in the car. I had totally blocked out everything she read to me. I put my trust and faith in the Lord.

Talk about being overwhelmed and speechless. Doctors are human they can make mistakes too. "If I truly had what she said, and was THAT far along in symptoms, I should be dead. Why, am I still alive?" I said confused.

They tried to comfort me in their own way. They agreed with me not to rest on what the medical report said. We all agreed that I should get another opinion because to us, God put doctors on earth for a reason. All I could do was smile. I wasn't going to worry about it. I had learned from my grandmother Arzola that worry is a sin. "Why worry about something that you have no control over," she would say.

It is what it is; worrying is not going to fix it or change it, but to trust God in prayer, because God has the last word. Esther and Michelle decide to take me to get something to eat at Cracker Barrel and to collect our thoughts after hearing such devastating news.

In the meantime, my symptoms had affected my ability to perform on my job efficiently. The doctor provided a letter for my supervisor stating: Dorothy, has fatigue and chronic itching that needs to be monitored under a doctor's care before I could consider returning her back to work.

Even though I wasn't able to go to work staying wasn't my cup of tea. I have worked for as long as I can remember, but this tormenting pain had become so intense that I could not even clean my home. The itching is severe unlike anything I have ever experienced and it is simply impossible to sit. My girlfriend Jewell Thomas and niece Anquette Henderson, came to the rescue.

I kept wearing my smile even though it had become obvious that I was itching more than I led on. It became more difficult to drive or simply stand still in one spot before my itching frenzy would be upon me in full force. It seemed like the itching was worst at night because it permits me to get any rest and peace.

One night I sat in the corner of my living room scratching my skin to the point that the itching overrode the itch. Suddenly, I felt as if invisible ants were crawling on the top of my skin every minute, every second! This was torment. All I had was God's word to stand on. I knew Him before the illness. I didn't call on His name just because something bad was happening to me. It was something I had always done, even in the good times. (We don't know God until something happens to ourselves or a loved one and then we call on Him). "The Lord is good, a strong hold in the day of troubles; and he knoweth them that trust in him" (Nahum 1:7).

> *The Lord is near to all who call upon Him,*
> *to all who call upon Him in truth.*
> Psalm 145:18-19

What may have been the most difficult to face was the fact that as an African American woman I had not known anyone who had an organ transplant in Michigan. It seemed taboo for African Americans to even think about receiving someone else's organs let alone signing a card to allow our organs to be donated upon our death. Some feel that if their organs are needed, the push to save their life in an accident will not be as urgent – not realizing that if needed someone's organs may help them in a time of need.

Some African Americans have such a spiritual outlook on life that we often neglect the signs that our bodies are giving us. We feel there is nothing prayer and faith won't cure. I believe whole-heartedly, that God has doctors in our lives to heal us through Him. While I was trying to understand everything that was happening to me, I asked God, "Why me?"

Although I tried to maintain a positive outlook, uplifting spiritual role model and forgive others. By trying to live righteous, have a sense of humor and not to disrespectful to others. Respect others feeling because none of us is perfect.

Whatever was going on with my physical body, I knew I had to speak to my body spiritually: This journey will begin a course; a test of faith, sickness must flee, fear and oppression have no power over me. God's word is my confession deep down in my heart and soul. There will be a liver waiting for me with my name on it because prayer changes things and I am healed. After all, you never know your strength of your faith until it is tested. For we walk by faith, not by sight (II Corinthians 5:7).

Today, I speak to this disease in my body–to confessing God's Word over my life, daily. "Speak healing, I am not sick." Perhaps through my trials of faith, I will run into some obstacle along the way to finish the course. I believe that I will overcome sickness and disease in Jesus' name. "I will win!"

> *And Jesus went about all the cities and villages, teaching in their synagogues, and preaching the gospel of the kingdom, and healing every sickness and every disease among the people.*
> Matthew 9:35

As time passed, my condition wasn't getting better. Some days I would feel fine, and then other days the torment returned. I begin to accept the fact I was ill – but I knew it would be only temporary. I continued going to the doctor but made an appointment for another opinion.

> *But he was wounded for our transgressions, he was bruised for our iniquities; the chastisement of our peace was upon him; and with his stripes we are healed.*
> Isaiah 53:5

This time my dad went with me to the doctor's appointment. It seemed as though the second doctor didn't help my case either. He began by saying that the itching was all in my head; not physical but mental! As he waited for the blood results I wondered why God was putting his child through this? Looking around the office, I noticed a pamphlet from the American Liver Foundation about alcohol and the liver. It reads, "What causes Cirrhosis?"

I learned that a long-term alcohol abuse and chronic hepatitis can cause cirrhosis. In children, the most frequent causes are biliary atresia, a disease that damages the bile ducts and neonatal hepatitis. Children with these diseases often receive liver transplants. Many adult patients who require liver transplants suffer from Primary Biliary Cirrhosis (PBC). It is known what causes this illness, but it is not any way related to alcohol consumption. Cirrhosis can also be cause by hereditary defects in iron or copper metabolism or prolonged exposure to toxins.

Cirrhosis vs. Liver Disease

Alcohol can cause liver disease, but it is only one of many causes and the risks vary on the amount and length of alcohol consumption.
There are more than 100 liver diseases. Known causes include viruses, hereditary defects, and actions to drugs and chemicals. Scientists are still investigating the causes for the most serious liver diseases.

When the doctor returned, he first apologized for telling me that my itching was all in my head. That still didn't help ease the fact that this diagnosis was the same as the first doctor's. My dad and I looked at each other shaking our heads.

"Surely, this report cannot be right?" Daddy said.

"Yes, I know," I said.

He replied, "You're not an alcohol drinker." My dad said, "Unless there something you not telling me, Dot?" We both giggled.

We tried to understand the medical report but were left dumbfounded. I went to one more physician and the verdict was unanimous. I had to face the facts and accept the truth that I had Primary Biliary Cirrhosis (PBC).

Since my life has changed so drastically since the year of 2000. The signs were there. I just didn't want to accept it. Even now, when I think about it, I couldn't believe how sick I was.

That Friday night, I had made plans to meet with my girlfriends to play pool at a restaurant called "Snicker's." When I was a no-show, Michelle called. I told her I was weak from not getting enough sleep.

Though deep down inside I should have told her I really needed to go to the hospital, but I told her that I would be okay. Another friend, Nathan Crite, called to check on me. I pushed off my weakness as a result of not having an appetite that day and needed to get some rest. He didn't believe me. He did not hear the one thing my voice always had – her bubbly self.

Nathan immediately called Esther telling her, "Something's not right with Dot. I spoke to her and she did not sound like herself. She was talking very soft, in a low-tone voice. I could hardly hear her. Something is wrong. She isn't her usual uplift or joyful self. You need to go check on her now."

Despite my defense that I had a doctor's appointment, I was to go for a more intensive examination on Monday. Esther was on her way to take me to the hospital. I tried to explained that I was referred to a doctor in Marshall, just about twenty minutes outside of Battle Creek on the I-94 corridor. There was no need to put up a fuss with Esther.

I had been in the house for a few days and needed a shower before I went anywhere. I walked doubled over to the bathroom, using the wall to hold me up along the way. I leaned against the shower wall trying not to fall as I washed up. When I heard Esther at the door, I tried my best to move as quickly as possible from the shower to the front door. While my mind wanted to move, my body could not. I stood there, frozen, wearing only a bath towel as tears ran down my face. Once I finally got to the door, Esther help me get dressed and rushed me to the emergency room at the Battle Creek Health System. Once again, she had been like the big sister I wished I had; a friend who had been there for me at my most vulnerable time.

"We're going to find out what is going on with you and you're not going back home until they do!" Esther said. I couldn't argue with her. I totally agreed! It was the right thing to do, if I want to feel better.

Once at the hospital my blood was drawn. The doctor admitted me. Esther didn't have to say anything more. God had my back by using Esther and her persistence to realize the severity of the situation. Later that evening, Esther had to catch a flight out of Detroit by 8:10 p.m., and she did not want to leave me alone. Esther called Katie Barnes to come quickly to the hospital to stay with me.

After Katie received the call, she hurried to the hospital. Then Esther called my parents to let them know I was in the hospital and not to worry that one of my girlfriends was there with me. Instead, of my mother waiting until the next day, she hurries to the hospital after she left work. It was not long before word spread that my situation was serious. Between my friend Katie, my family and coworkers, they kept me encouraged through visits and prayer.

The next morning, Mother Georgia Howard came to visit me with a beautiful red rose in a vase to brighten my room. She prayed for me with her pleasant smile until it was time for her to leave. I wanted her to stay with me a little longer, because she always shows me Jesus' love.

(Later, into my journey, I had went to visit mother Howard. I begin extreme itching all over my body. I felt so embarrassed. But mother Howard understood my condition and we continue to enjoy one another's company. The next day, there was a surprise wooden backscratcher left in my mailbox from mother Howard. "Thank-you, mother Howard, I love you." It surely came in good used.) Although, I was given a medication called, 'Questran' to help stop the itching, it didn't work!

All throughout the night, the itching was so unbearable that I asked the Lord, "If He wanted to call me home tonight, I understood." At the same time, I wanted to be there for my grandchildren to tell them about a man named Jesus as my grandmother told me when I was a child. But I just could not stand the sickness and nausea anymore. That night was rough. I could not stand the vomiting anymore. I just wanted to go home—not heaven, yet!

(I was truly blessed to have two loving grandmothers who loved the Lord. Their memories will always be in my heart, forever. There is nothing like having a relationship with your grandmothers. Today, I missed them both very much. You never realize how much you miss someone when something happens or they no longer here with us.)

The comfort of visitors did help at least ease my mind. The visitor's list was long which included family, friends and church members. I greeted each of them with a smile; that was the least I could do under the circumstances. Phone calls, cards, visitor's, and my greetings sent by others continued to roll in. I was blessed to be touch by so many people that cared about me.

After two weeks in the hospital, doctors said my liver was so damaged that they didn't expect me to live much longer. I thanked God that I was a Christian and waited on Him to have the last word. I was sent home with plans to follow-up with another doctor in a few weeks for specifically prescribed medication needed to comfort me. I knew in my heart, God had more for me to do here on earth and this would be just one of the trials He would bring me through.

When I was discharged from the Battle Creek Health System, I went home weighing only 90 pounds. Michelle didn't want me to be alone, so she felt it was best that I stay with her for a while. She took the time to give me a bath, wash my hair, prepare meals and give me my medication on time; all this while taking care of her own family. I thank God for my best friend for being a part of my life and supporting me with genuine love.

One day while Michelle was at work, her coworker, George Gray asked, "How is Dot doing?"

At that moment, Michelle looked at him and broke down in tears as she cried on his shoulder. (No one wants to see anyone sick or helpless. Especially, when tragedy strikes and it will. It can be devastating when the person has always been considered very healthy; then to see sickness and suffering in their lives. Yes, it can bring sadness to one's heart.) After staying with Michelle for two weeks, I knew it was time for me return back home, alone.

Because of the medication the doctor prescribed, I could not keep food on my stomach and I was continually vomiting. I never had taken any type of medication until I became ill. I have always been a healthy person. It seemed as if the medications weren't working at all! Because of my nausea, I was not able to go to the pharmacy any longer. I felt hopeless and scared.

My dad and mother had to go back and forth to the pharmacy to pick-up my prescriptions. My mother worked second shift at Post Cereal so she was able to pick-up medicine before heading to work. She always told me how much she loves me and gave me a hug. At times, I could see her pain of the fear that she could be losing a child. I couldn't imagine, as a mother, having to prepare for the worst or pray that my daughter be healed.

One day my dad saw how weak I was. He gently held me in his arms and I sobbed quietly all over his jacket. He reached in this jacket pocket and handed me a handkerchief to blow my nose. My dad knew all I needed was a loving hug to comfort me.

He said, "Dot, you my oldest daughter, this too shall pass. Trouble don't last always. You have to believe that you are going to get better and it's going to alright in Jesus' name."

All I could do was smile. When I tried to return his handkerchief, he said, "That's okay baby, why don't you keep it for now!" My dad and I both laughed.

I knew I could count on both my parents, but I could not stand the idea of putting wear and tear on them for my sake. So, I had to put aside my pride and ask others such as my daughter, sister, Ola and my dearest friends to pitch in.

One day I called Ola to see if she could pick up my prescriptions from the pharmacy. As she brought the medication into the house, I could see her pain. She was quiet as she handed me the bottle of medication. She asks me how I was doing. My reply, "I'm hanging in there patiently and waiting on the manifestation of God to heal me."

She said, "I heard that," as she smiled. She embraced me with a big hug and let me know how much she loved me.

The next day, my best girl, Esther stopped by the house to check on me. I still had been unable to keep any food down. Esther had to go to the pharmacy to pick up another prescription. She could see me holding back tears of hopelessness. I was tired of experiencing all the different types of medicines that the doctor prescribed. I felt I was being used as a guinea pig as I prayed that the right medicine would adjust to my body, and help avoid the vomiting.

"It is going to be alright, we're going to find the right medicine to help you with your condition," Esther said. "It will take to get in your system and get adjusted to you. Dot, have faith, and know that the battle is not yours, it's the Lord's." She hugged me and we both smiled.

"Yes, I have faith and I am strong; but there has been time I felt weak because I have had to lean on everyone for help," I told her. "And that is not me, or fair to anyone! I don't want anyone to feel sorry for me. It's hard to wake up one day, and to see how quickly your whole life can change in ways that you couldn't have imagined."

"You don't understand. Nobody is complaining!" Esther said, "Snapped out of it! So, please stop feeling sad or sorry for yourself and let everyone that loves you, care FOR you, and let us deal with the situation. We are here to help you. So get a grip! That is why God put friends in our path. Therefore, when something does happen we are here to be a blessing to each other. Now show me that smile?"

Later that evening Esther went home. I started to feel a little better and was able to keep food down with the medication that she had delivered. This was the right one! All I could say was, "Thank you Lord."

> *The Lord will give strength unto his people; the Lord will bless his people with peace.*
> Psalm 29:11

My mother-in-law, Doris Dearring, was one of those who always kept in contact with me throughout my illness. She would send a card, telephone me and come from Detroit to visit with her daughter, Trivia and daughter-in-law, Deborah Dearring.

One evening my sister-in-law, Yvette Dearring, makes a trip from California to Detroit and asked if I could come to see her. I asked my daughter, Nicole to drive me there. It was delightful and joyful time as we ate and took photos together with the virtuous, beautiful, and radiant Dearring women of God.

Throughout my illness, I had so many visitors including my ex-husband and his fiancée, Robin. When I first met Robin, we connected as spiritual sisters as if we had known one another all our lives.

That the trial of your faith, being much more precious than of gold that perisheth, though it be tried with fire, might be found unto praise and honour and glory at the appearing of Jesus Christ.
Whom having not seen, ye love; in whom, though now ye see him not, yet believing, ye rejoice with joy unspeakable and full of glory.
I Peter 1:7-8

On August 25, 2001, Dad drove me to the doctor's office to meet Dr. Pasricha whose review of me was the following recanted in a Letter of Consultation: *After a referral from R.C. Bhan, M.D.

Reason for consultation: This patient was consulted today at the request of Dr. Bhan for evaluation of liver failure and jaundice.

History: The patient is 45-year-old, Black female who states she was in pretty good health until approximately 3 or 4 weeks ago when she started itching (on her job) – really all over her body, legs, arms, abdomen, and it had become somewhat uncontrollable.

She saw her regular doctor and about three weeks ago was diagnosed with liver failure. She also was diagnosed with Mono by blood test. The itching got worse today and she also had some nonspecific nausea, and she subsequently was admitted with diagnosed liver failure. She says she has not been confused at all or is she making it up in her head; nor has she had any vomiting but the nausea is mild and only when the itching is going on.

There is no abdominal discomfort, dysphagia, odynophagia or early satiety. No heartburn – type symptoms. No melena, hematochezia, diarrhea, constipation, or any clay colored stools. Her urine has been a normal color and there has been no dysuria or hematuria. She does not smoke or drink. She does not know of an exposure to anyone with hepatitis. There has been no history any type of intravenous drug abuse, tattoos, or illicit drug abuse such as cocaine abuse. She has never had any blood transfusions. She denies any abdominal trauma.

Medications: She takes no routine medications except for multivitamins at times. She has also been on treatment with Benadryl and Pepcid here in the hospital.

Allergies: Codeine

Family History: The family history is not significant for any types of gallbladder disease, liver disease, or cancer. She believes it's on her mother's side there–her grandmother's sister (Aunt Tim Geer) had ovarian cancer.

Recommendations: At this time I recommend starting Questan – it may help her itching and she understands that it may not, however, I want to at least give it a try. Please check ceruloplasmin, cooper, iron, TIBC and ferritin, ANA as well as anti-smooth muscle antibody, anti-mitochomdrial antibody, and alpha-1 antitrypsin level.

Patient understands the fact that her prothrombin is normal and means that her liver is working but simply irritated and we need to go out in and see what is going on to cause this process and that is why we are checking multiple liver tests and CAT scans have been done to check for any inter-abdominal malignancies playing a role in this situation such as lymphoma which can present with these liver function abnormalities.

Signature: S.P.Pasricha, M.D

September 19, 2001

Referred by: Dr. Bhan: Primary Phys: Dr. Chauvin

Reason for Office Visit: Intrahepatic cholestasis - positive monospot serology, positive primary Biliary cirrhosis serology (antimitochondrial antibody was positive).

Brief History: Dorothy Dearring follows up today with her father. Unfortunately, she has had some itching. She does not think the Questran is helping at all and I have asked her to stop the Questran. The itching may have gotten a little worse recently. She denies any nausea or vomiting. No fatigue and no increasing jaundice. No major abdominal pain–occasionally on the right side but nothing major.

Review of Systems: No chest pain, palpitations, wheezing or shortness of breath. Physical Examination: Physical examination reveals blood pressure is 140/80, pulse of 100, respiratory rate 20. She weighs 119 pounds. Her lungs were clear to auscultation and percussion. Abdomen was soft, non-distended and non-tender. No organomegaly or masses. Sclerae were somewhat icteric. Extremities had no cyanosis, clubbing or edema. There were some excoriations noted. She was alert and oriented X3. No asterixis.

Data Base: I don't have CT scan and ultrasound results from when she was in hospital but apparently they showed no ductal dilatation and we need to get copies for our records. In other words, nothing significant was seen to explain her cholestasis. She had a positive monospot serology on two occasions but this should not cause all these problems. Her alkaline phosphatase is high at 1620, SGOT 184, SGPT 187, total bilirubin 4.4, BUN 11, creatinine 1.0.

Her Hepatitis A antibody IgM was negative. Hepatitis B surface antigen was negative. Hepatitis C antibody was negative. Her ANA was positive at 1:160, sedimentation rate 86 which is elevated, anti-smooth muscle antibody less than 1:20. Her antimitochondrial antibody was 1:640.

Alpha-1 antitrypsin level was normal at 179. Her iron was 115, TIBC 342, ferritin 1302.6, copper 2206, which is elevated; ceruloplasmin was 70.6 which are elevated. Alpha fetoprotein was 2.0. Her ammonia level was elevated at 40. Her Tylenol level was less than 1.0. CMV 1gG was greater than 299. Prothrombin time was 11.3 on 08/27/2001. Hemoglobin was 12.7, platelet count 296,000, white blood cell count 5,600. Hepatitis B surface antibody was negative also.

Impression: Primary Biliary Cirrhosis – I gave the patient a handout to read on what is primary biliary cirrhosis (PBC) regard to the disease. She understands that primary Biliary cirrhosis is granulomatous destruction of the small Intrahepatic bile ducts which can lead to Intrahepatic cholestasis with significant pruritus as well as cirrhosis of the liver itself.

Unfortunately, I don't have the exact CT scan and ultrasound reports at this time but I understand these are normal as far as any ductal dilatation is concerned. She understands that primary biliary cirrhosis has no known cause – it was nothing she did to get this.

There is not a very good treatment out there, although Actigall has had some use in prolonged survival of some patients. She is having a lot of itching right now and her bilirubin is slightly elevates and I think it is important that we get her involved with a transplant center because I have a feeling she is going to need a transplant in the future.

We also want get a liver biopsy on her staging. Elevated ANA–elevated ANA and sedimentation rate can sometimes be seen in people with PBC. Her anti-smooth muscle antibody was negative. History of positive monospot – I don't think this is anything that significant. Perhaps she had two things going on at once. History of itching and nausea–the nausea is better. The itching/pruritus is more than likely due to her Intrahepatic cholestasis. Family history of ovarian cancer– on her mother's side and diabetes–on both side of her family. The patient may need evaluation in the future. Increased liver function tests–more than likely secondary to #1.

Recommendations: I have asked her to increase her Actigall 600 mg b.i.d. Discontinue Questran as it has not been helping much. Her primary care doctor put her on Ativan and Benadryl and she is to continue these. We need to do a Liver Biopsy on her. She understands the indications, risks, complications, benefits, alternatives, as well as limitations in this regard. The ways of doing it include ultra- sound-guided, CT-guided, laparoscopic, open or percutaneously.

At this time, she is somewhat large around the mid body and I cannot get good landmarks to do it pertinaciously. I think we need to do an ultra-sound, and she agreed. This scheduled for next week. We need to send her to a transplant center. Therefore, they decided to send her to University of Michigan, for evaluation of primary Biliary cirrhosis and itching. Follow-up on 10/10/2001. Further recommendations depending on how she does.

SPP/dmk Sunil P. Pasericha, M.D.

If you can believe, all things are possible to him that believeth.

Mark 9:23

Chapter 4

IN THE MEANTIME

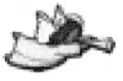

2001

I was scheduled to have an Ultrasound Guide Needle biopsy. My girlfriend, Pat Doggett, planned to fly in from Atlanta, Georgia that weekend to be with me in the morning before the procedure. She stayed at my home to help prepare meals and clean while taking care of me. It was good to talk and laugh, even if I had to do most of it in bed.

Esther picked us up on the day of the procedure and stayed with us until I waited to be seen. While waiting we saw a coworker from my job who, said he heard that I was dying because of my liver failure. We all looked in shock as the words rolled out of his mouth so matter-of-factly. My girlfriends were upset at his audacity and the rumor that apparently had been spreading around town.

Here I am sitting here in the hospital waiting room ready to get a biopsy and I was already being pronounced dead! All I could do was smile, then laugh. As I prepared for my procedure my neighbor, Val Mabry, and my Bishop's wife, Letha Smith, came to surprise me. I felt so special. The First Lady Letha laid her healing hands upon my right upper abdomen in the direction of my liver.

At the same time, Val laid her hands upon my forehead as they both prayed for a positive outcome. They both gave me a Holy kiss and hug before they left. Esther and Pat continued to wait for me in the waiting area. I am so grateful and blessed to have beautiful, loving friends placed in my path by God.

Before the biopsy, the diagnosis of Primary Biliary Cirrhosis (PBC) is based on several pieces of information. Itching and fatigue alert the physician that bile ducts may be damaged. As previously, mentioned, high levels of certain liver enzymes in the blood are important clues.

Probably the most important laboratory test is one for mitochondrial antibodies. Mitochondria are the energy sources within cells.

For unknown reasons, a protein antibody develops against them in 95 percent of PBC cases. The physician must look at the whole picture to make the diagnosis of PBC. Often the physician x-rays the bile ducts to rule out other causes of obstruction. This x-ray, called an ERCP, is performed under light sedation. A flexible endoscope is inserted through the stomach and then into the small intestine.

A thin tube is placed through the scope into the bile ducts, and dye is injected to highlight the bile ducts on the x-ray. As the disease progresses, a liver biopsy is needed to determine how much damage has occurred. Under local anesthesia, a slender needle inserted through the right lower chest to extract a small piece of liver for microscopic analysis.

The nurse rolled me to the radiology department. (I took a deep breath and said a silent prayer.) The risks and benefits of the liver biopsy were explained to the patient who consented. The skin overlying the left anterior approach to the liver was prepped and draped in the usual sterile fashion. One percent Lidocaine was used for local anesthesia. Under ultrasound guidance, a 19-gauge needle was inserted into the liver and several biopsies were obtained and placed in formal in without complication.

As the procedure continues, I looked above knowing God was right there with me. The nurse who assisted the doctor squeezed my hand; I squeeze back. This was the first procedure that I had to experience fully awake. When it was over the Pathology consultation submitted the report on a liver biopsy tissue and forward the information to University of Michigan in Ann Arbor Michigan.

The report read:

History: Primary Biliary Cirrhosis

Specimen(s) Submitted: A liver biopsy

Tissue Gross Description: In Formalin labeled "liver biopsy."

Microscopic Description: The specimen consists of thin needle biopsy of liver. Due to the small caliber of the biopsy, definitive diagnosis is not possible. Nevertheless, the portal tracts are expanded by lymphocytes and some histiocytes. There is some piecemeal necrosis.

There is some rare bile duct damage but definitive granulomas are not seen. A rare focus of acute inflammation is also identified. The iron stain is negative for iron. The reticulin stain shows a nonspecific increase in reticulin. The trichrome stain shows increased and fibrous connective tissue primarily around the portal tracts but also extending into the lobules.

Comment: It is noted that the patient's anti-mitochondrial antibody is increased and the copper levels are also greatly increased. It is also noted that the patient is negative for viral hepatitis. The overall picture therefore, is consistent with Primary Biliary Cirrhosis, stage II. This case was reviewed by Dr. Flynn and Myers who agree with the diagnosis.

On October 10, 2001, my dad took me to see Dr. Sunil P. Pasricha, M.D., who explained that my condition wasn't getting any better. By the time we left the office, we both were more confused. I trusted God to heal me. I heard what the doctor said, but that did not mean I had to receive it.

I was referred to a doctor at University of Michigan Medical Center in Ann Arbor, MI. The doctors in Battle Creek had done all they could.

Dr. Pasricha, forward this to the University of Michigan:

Dear Doctors,

This is a letter of introduction to Dorothy Dearring. She is a pleasant 45-year old black female whose care I first became involved with on August 25, 2001. I was asked to see to her because of jaundice. Her ultrasound of the abdomen as normal without any ductal dilatation.

The gallbladder was also unremarkable as well as the Liver. ACT scan of the abdomen and pelvis was also done and both were unremarkable. I suspect she has Intrahepatic cholestasis – her alkaline phosphatase was about 1620 with an SGOT of 184 and SGPT of 187. Total was 4.4. Prothrombin time was normal at 11.8. An evaluation was done to find the cause of this Intrahepatic cholestasis and hepatitis A, B, and C serologies were unremarkable.

Previously a monospot was positive and this was repeated again three weeks prior to when I saw her. I repeated it again and it was still positive. Other important labs include an ANA of 1:160, which is elevated at our hospital. Sedimentation rate was elevated at 86 but her anti-smooth muscle antibody was less than 1:20. Her anti- mitochondrial antibody was quite elevated in 1:640.

Her copper was 2206, which is quite elevated at our institution with a ceruloplasmin of 70.6. Her ferritin were elevated at 1302.6, iron 115 and TIBC 342 (both of these are normal). Alpha-1 antitrypsin level was 170. Her Tylenol level was normal at 4 but ammonia was elevated one time at 40. Eventually quantitative immunoglobulins were done and her 1gM was elevated at 378 with an IgG elevated in 1970 and 1gA of 187, which is normal at our hospital.

An ultrasound-guided liver biopsy was done and this was suggestive of stage-II primary Biliary cirrhosis–it was suggestive of but not completely diagnostic of it, according to our pathologist (the patient was instructed to take the actual liver biopsy sides to your office when she sees you).

The main problem is that she is having itching and we have tried Questran up to 4gm q.i.d. without much relief, and she stopped this. She is on URSO at 600 mg b.i.d. without much relief either. Today I saw her in the office and I am going to start her on rifampicin 300mg b.i.d. in hopes that this will help her. We also may possibly send her to a tanning booth for UV exposure in the future. Because of her clinical situation, I thought it would be appropriate for her to come and see you at the University of Michigan for further evaluation as far as the itching and anything else we can do about her primary Biliary cirrhosis.

Obviously, she may need a transplant in the future and I think it is important that we get her involved at your institution now rather than later on. She has an appointment to see you on November 14, 2001, and hopefully you can help her out. In the meantime, I have also instructed the patient to take vitamin D and calcium. If you have any questions, please do not hesitate to contact me.

Sincerely,
Sunil P. Pasricha, MD

I was referred to Dr. Jorge A. Marrero's, office on November 14, 2001, at the University of Michigan Hospital in Ann Arbor. He was pleasant, had a joyful spirit, and a caring heart. We instantly connected. It was a world of difference compared to Battle Creek Health System. At the same time, I had never seen so many sick people in one place. It was times like these when I realized that there is always someone who is worse off than you. The spirit of sickness and pain were in the atmosphere and prayed for the spirit of healing to outweigh the spirit of sickness.

I was feeling desperate to getting my life back to being the person I used to be—healthy. This disease is still very new to me, but I had to wait on God and deal with it temporarily. As with material prosperity, good health is not a sign of spirituality or divine favor. Neither is sickness necessarily a sign of sin, unbelief, or God's displeasure. The key is to believe God at His word, which says, And the Lord will take away from you all sickness, and will afflict you with none of the terrible diseases of Egypt which you known, but will lay them on all those who hate you (Deuteronomy 7:15). We need to believe God's Word and avoid making judgment with our limited understanding regarding others.

After keeping all appointments, I had to keep hope alive in my heart. Continually, I believed God's word; that He would make a way for me no matter what the doctors said. I remember reading about when Jesus went out about all of Galilee teaching in their synagogues, preaching the gospel of the kingdom, and healing all the manner of sickness and all manner of disease among the people.

And His fame went throughout all Syria: and they brought unto Him all sick people that were taken with divers diseases and torments, and those which were possessed with devils, and those which were lunatic, and those that had palsy; and he healed them.
Matthew 4:24

As I read the scripture, I thought of the awful torment an illness can bring to the human physical body, especially when you have no control to stop it. I continued to attend Sunday church and Wednesday night Bible Study. I knew there was no place in my life for a pity-party, only prayer. It is what it is, why stress over the circumstance when you cannot change it.

For more than a year, my physical torment had become mental. It was causing me to become frustrated and fatigue; I had swelling ankles, my skin easily bruised, and constant itching all over my entire body. I had thought of suicide – but I refuse to put that burden on the people who I loved.

Through it all, I had to show the world that my talk of Jesus' love was not just words. He does exist! I want the world to know, that God lives in me and would help me get through this trial. I had to be a witness through my testimony of healing. I made up my mind that I shall live and not die. What the devil meant for evil, God meant it for good. Regardless, of my circumstance or situation I knew I had to go THROUGH this so I could give all the glory to God.

And he that searcheth the hearts knoweth what is the mind of the Spirit, because he maketh intercession for the saints according to the will of God. And we know that all things work together for good to them that love God, to them who are the called according to his purpose.
Romans 8:27-28

December 2001

Reason For Office Visit/Chief Complaint: Intrahepatic cholestasis, primary biliary cirrhosis.

Brief History: Ms. Dorothy Dearring follows up today and is doing better.

I started her on rifampin 300 mg b.i.d. and her itching has improved. The University of Michigan switched her Actigall to URSO 250 mg p.o.t.i.d. She had some problems with nonspecific nausea and was put on Protonix every day. She was having headaches she does not think the Protonix made the headaches any worse. She has not started any calcium or vitamin D at this time. She denies any dysphagia or early satiety. No nausea or vomiting right now. No diarrhea, constipation, melena or hematochezia. She has not had any blood loss at all. Her itching has not improved.

Physical Examination: Physical examination reveals blood pressure is 110/72, pulse of 84, respiratory rate 20. She weighs 138 pounds. Her lungs were clear to auscultation and percussion. Abdomen was soft, non-distended and non-tender. Extremities had no edema.

She understands what primary biliary cirrhosis is – it is granulomatous destruction of the bile ducts which can lead to cirrhosis of the liver. It can also cause some osteopenia and osteoporosis and that is why we want to get her on some calcium and vitamin D.

Impression:

1. Primary biliary cirrhosis–she is in an early stage. There is no obvious cirrhosis on liver biopsy but there is profound ductopenia.

2. History of positive monospot–again, I think this is not the cause of any of her problems, however, it may have made things worse.

3. History of nausea–better.

4. History of increased liver function tests – secondary to #1.

Recommendations:
1. Hemoccult testing x3.
2. Repeat CBC and comprehensive medical panel – it has been about a month since the last time.
3. Follow up in about a month. An appointment is made for January 10, 2002. Hold off on any type of tanning booth light therapy–this may make her photo sensitivity worse but it also may make the itching better. We are going to hold off this time since she has done better with the combination of URSO and rifampin.

SPP/dmk

2002

Two years have passed. My life has been flipped-turned upside down by this disease. As time seems to pass, my condition was not getting better but it was not getting worse, either. But I continued to press my way to do my daily routine. There was no way I was going to quit! My fresh and my heart faileth: but God is the strength of my heart and my portion forever (Psalm 73:26).

I remember reading cirrhosis can cause liver failure and other serious problems. In the early stages of the disease, the main problem caused by PBC is the build-up of substances in the liver and bloodstream. The doctors stated my bile ducts were blocked or missing and the flow of bile was restricted. There was no way for my liver to filter or break down the toxins chemicals, dead blood and bacteria through the body.

This is a disease in which the body's immune system attacks the normal components, or cells, of the liver and causes inflammation and liver damage. The hardest test of my circumstance was in the mist of the midnight hour. The doctor prescribed Ambien to help me sleep. The sleeping pill was only a temporary fix that would help physical and emotionally, and allow me to get some peace.

The itching had other side effects such as dryness, rash of redness, which appeared on my body, and aches that were painful to the skin and body. Talk about woe is me! But there was no time to complain or feel sorry for myself. I had to use a variety of skin medications and treatments—which many of them didn't work.

Because the University of Michigan is a teaching hospital, the physicians themselves do a great job in explaining to patients their illness. The doctor explained that the Primary Biliary Cirrhosis (PBC) of the liver could have occurred in my body when I was a child and was just coming to surface. They explained that babies sometime develop cirrhosis as a result of Billiard Artesia, a condition in which the bile ducts are closed or missing at birth. Usually an individual with liver disease can develop more serious complications and may not live past six years. Liver transplantation is usually an option for patients with liver failure and the outcome is 70 percent survival at seven years. During the first two months in Ann Arbor, Dr. Jorge Marrero requested I have some family members or friends to come and listen to a young lady speak about her own liver transplant.

My parents, stepmother, Ethel, girlfriends, Esther Harden and Jeanette Payne, piled into my father's van to hear the presentation in Ann Arbor. For more than two years, they all had been by my side, every step of the way.

The road to Ann Arbor however, would detour after my insurance coverage would only pay 70 percent of my medical bill for a transplant. We learned there was a hospital that would do the transplant and would qualify for 100 percent coverage by my insurance. Unfortunately, I hated to leave Dr. Jorge Marrero, who I had grown so fond of; it was time to switch our driving from I-94 East, to I-94 West...to Chicago.

But my God shall supply all your need according to his riches in glory by Christ Jesus.

Philippians 4:19

Chapter 5

THE WAIT

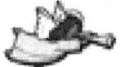

2003

Chicago is less than three hours from Battle Creek; however, I had never been there. My desire had always been to visit a taping of the *Oprah Winfrey Show*, then visit Johnson Publishing Company, the creators of the iconic *Ebony* and *Jet* magazines. Instead, my visits to Chicago would be strictly to receive treatments at Northwestern Memorial Hospital, with the goal of getting a new liver.

My connection to the hospital also puts me one step closer to healing. On our first day to the Windy City, my dad drove to I-94 East on to exit I-55 North and then to Lake Shore Drive South towards the marvelously tall building called Northwestern Memorial Hospital. There I would meet the evaluation team. I had to meet with a hepatologist, liver surgeon, social worker, nutritionist, financial coordinator, psychiatrist, medical librarian, pre-liver transplant nurse coordinators and clinical coordinators.

The plan: I would receive initial blood work, transplant work order, heart evaluation (echo and stress test), lung evaluation pulmonary function test, and additional tests/procedures in the event any illness or complications would arise. This required that I return for follow-up appointments and comply with the prescribed medications, procedures and tests. If I did not show up for the appointments, tests or procedures, etc., I could be put on a transplant hold and even be removed from the transplant waiting list.

The timing: The transplant could influence its success yet; proper timing is not easy to determine. The best timing for a transplant is before you become severely ill and before the diseased liver causes serious complications that could affect recovery. Physicians who specialize in treating liver disorders (hepatologists and transplant surgeons) define the urgency for each patient's transplant.

The matching: The size of the liver and blood type (positive or negative doesn't matter) is crucial in a liver transplant. Blood Group O is the universal donor and O can only use O liver; Blood Group A can use O or A liver; Blood Group B can use O or B liver; Blood Group AB (the universal acceptor), AB can use O, A, or B liver.

The time and date of a liver match could not be predicted. In the meantime, the transplant teams continued to monitor my condition. If my health got worse, I would require hospitalization for management of my liver condition. The waiting period was difficult and doctors encourage me to talk to family's members, friends and even clergy about any anxieties or fears. Through it all, I was told to maintain as much of a routine lifestyle as possible, and to just wait.

But they that wait upon the Lord shall renew their strength; they shall mount up with wings as eagles; they shall run, and not weary; and they shall walk, and not faint.
Isaiah 40:31

On August 27, 2003, I received a letter from the Kovler Organ Transplant Center, which read:

Dear Ms. Dorothy Dearring:

We would like to inform you that you have been placed on the liver transplant wait list. We have reviewed your medical records, all of the information from your initial evaluation visit, and as well as the results of your transplant work up.

At present there does not appear to be any medical or other contra indications toward transplantation. Therefore, your case was presented and reviewed by the multidisciplinary transplant committee and they determined you as a good potential candidate for a liver transplantation. To remain a liver transplant candidate, you will be required to comply with the physicians, transplant nurse coordinator and rules of the Northwestern Liver Transplant Program or you will be removed from the liver transplant waiting list. The rules included: no non-prescribed medications (drugs) or alcohol use, must return to the liver transplant clinic for follow-up visits when instructed, and must comply with all of the requests and orders from the physicians and transplant nurse coordinators.

You must also contact the financial (insurance) coordinator if there is any change in your insurance or your insurance coverage. All of us on the Liver Transplant Team appreciate the opportunity to take part in your medical care.

Sincerely yours,

Michael Abecassis M.D. Associate Professor of Surgery,
Director of Liver Transplantation

At this point in my life, there was no turning back. I knew God had my back and I loudly professed, "I am healed, I am healed, I am healed in Jesus' Name!" I was determined, as a Christian woman, to stay strong, have courage, believe in God's word, pray, keep the faith, continue to press, never to give up, and have a will to live. No matter what my outward appearance showed (bruises, itching and sores) or how I was feeling inside, I knew God's grace was keeping me.

Every day was a struggle but I had to speak to my spiritual self and continue to believe in a miracle. I spoke healing to myself while in the shower, in the elevator, driving to work, at my desk–everywhere. I'm taking back everything the Devil stole from me!

My friend from church, Antoinette Hardeman, came to my home and brought me scriptures based on healing and to post them around the home for me to meditate by speaking it to existing; where our faith may be tested and therefore, through trials, and be strengthened. I placed them on my bathroom wall and bedroom mirror where they be the first thing I see each morning. I surrounded myself daily with encouraging and healing scriptures to read out loudly.

> *Wait on the Lord: be of good courage, and he shall strengthen thine heart: wait, I say, on the Lord.*
> Psalm 27:14

> *I can do all things through Christ, which strengthened me.*
> Philippians 4:13

> *I shall not die, but live and declare the works of the Lord.*
> Psalm 118:17

> *So then faith cometh by hearing, and hearing by the word of God.*
> Romans 10:17

> *And the Lord direct your heart into love of God, and into the patient waiting for Christ.*
> 2 Thessalonians 3:5

> *Wherefore take unto you the whole armor of God, that ye may be able to withstand in the evil day, and having done all, to stand.*
> Ephesians 6:13

Through all of the doctor visit, motivation from family and dearest friends and my own attempts at staying encouraged, when it came down to it, I simply had to wait on the Lord. Unfortunately, waiting was the hardest part throughout this journey. I felt like I was holding every breath in my body and I was waiting to exhale. Waiting and hoping to receive the call that would announce a liver was ready, was literally like being on hold on God's phone line.

Organ transplant candidates who have family members who are eligible donors are truly lucky. They do not have to wait on a list and can go straight into surgery. The rest of us have to cope with the waiting, which is often more stressful than the ailment itself. For those whose lives are teetering between life and death as they wait an organ, the wait can be unbearable.

Wait means, to remain inactive or stay in one spot until something anticipated occurs. I had no choice but to wait on God's timing for my healing. God's perfect timing is not ours. I continually asked myself, *When am I going to get my new liver?* It was useless. (When we try to take matters into our own hands and help God out, we get in trouble.) I simply had to wait, and be quiet!

Waiting was not as stressful as long as I was physically able to work. Working gave me a chance to keep my mind off my condition. But I seemed to get exhausted with just the slightest of activity. I had to keep telling myself that I had to learn to live with my condition, temporary.

There was many times I phoned my cousin Kathy Mabry, and we continue to hang out together whenever I had a good day. Laying in bed was not something I like to do. At times, it could be distressful and depressing. I am a woman who likes to get up, and go and enjoy life. Weeping may endure for a night, but I'm glad that I still have joy!

For his anger endureth but a moment; in favour is life: weeping may endure for a night, but joy cometh in the morning.
Psalm 30:5

One day, I supposed to meet Kathy at her house to spend some "girl time" when suddenly I was falling asleep behind the sterling wheel of my automobile in Big Lots parking lot. While Kathy was waiting on me, she became concerned and uncomfortable when I hadn't returned her calls.

She knew it was not like me not to phone her back. I soon was awakened by a loud horn. I quickly ran to a telephone booth to phone Kathy to let her know how sorry I was and I was all right. Kathy said, "Good, I am glad that you're OK." For some reason I could not keep my eyelids open. Even though we never made it to the mall, we detoured to a Sprint store to buy me a cellphone.

Michelle often plans events where she invited friends and coworkers for an evening of music with a musician named, Yancyy of Detroit. On December 27, 2003, she married her handsome knight and shining amour, Ronnie Franklin. The wedding was at Stouffer's Hotel in downtown Battle Creek, and Yancyy was there to perform. The evening was luxurious and beautifully decorated with lovely flowers and an atmosphere of romance. Michelle's two lovely daughters, Bianca and Aja Smith were her maids of honor. Enjoying the moments–of love and seeing two wonderful people truly in love, forever!

I have been used of living alone and doing for myself. It gave me the perfect opportunity to be in tune with God since my divorce. I was living the good life as a Christian woman. "The Lord is good unto them that wait for him, to the soul that seeketh him" (Lamentation 3:25).

I have never been one to depend on others to help drive me to appointments, clean my house–all the things I used to do with ease–took away my independence. What I could control was keeping my body ready the transplant. I continued to exercise (when I had the strength and energy) by walking and talking to Jesus with every step of faith. I knew that the healthier I was at the time of the surgery the more successful the transplant would be.

I decided to learn as much as I could about a liver transplantation. When I began to understand what I going through and what to expect, it eased so much anxiety. I went on the Internet website to collect important information on liver disease. At times, the information could be overwhelming.

Thoughts of suicide kept running through my mind. I continued to rebuke the devil and proclaim, "I will live and not die, in Jesus' Name!" I held on to my favorite scriptures close to my heart: "Now faith is the substance of things hoped for, the evidence of things not seen" (Hebrews 11:1).

One of my neighbors, Dorothy People, shared healing messages by other pastors through the tapes she let me used. Another friend from church, Darlene Morris, brought me spiritual tapes also of healing messages by our Bishop Hugh D. Smith, Jr., and Rev. Creflo Dollar. My desire to read the Bible became a challenge as I constantly itching, then chronic fatigue, sat in. Mother Cherrie Williams let me listen to her, "King James complete Bible on audio tape." That way I could continue to hear God's word.

My neighbors and friends continue to show their love and support by bringing me food, even taking my trash cart to the curb or shoveling my driveway. I tried to maintain as much normalcy as possible by attending wedding, church banquets, performing at poetry jam and baking cakes for graduations. Thinking positively and not allowing negativity to weigh me down was a key to remain healthy inside. Through it all, I knew God was working on the inside of me.

In the past, I did my best to be independent. Over the past three years, I had been humbled in so many ways. I had to learn to let others help me and swallow my pride. I could no longer be embarrassed or ashamed by my illness. I needed a transplant because I was very sick. Once I receive the transplant, I knew I could get back to doing more for myself. At the same time, I could never forget those who helped and forever, remember to bless them back in any way I could.

Some people will not accept Christ as their personal savior, because they don't want to change their ways. But you can't be healed or changed by holding onto sinful ways and expecting God to hear your prayers. Pride is a sin, and not wanting to relinquish it could lead to unanswered prayers.

Jesus answered and said unto him, Verily, verily, I say unto thee, Except a man be born again, he cannot see the kingdom of God.
John 3:3

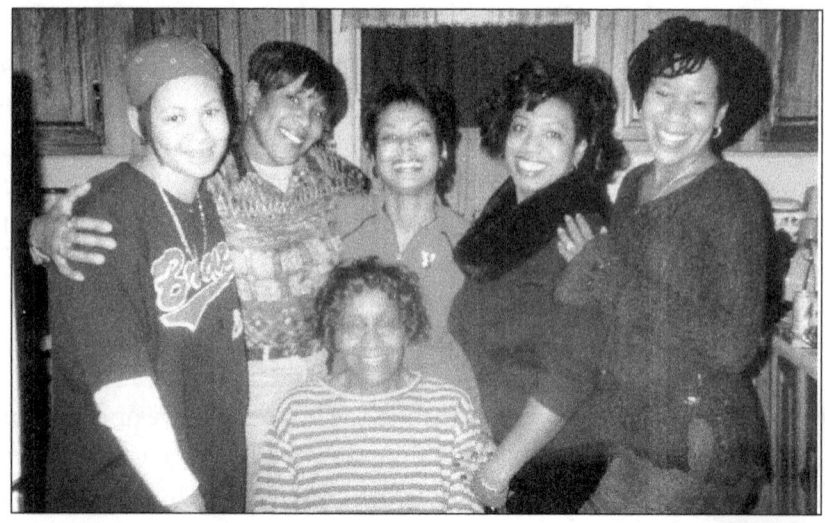
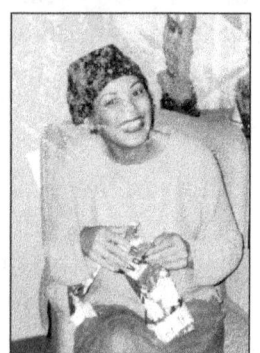
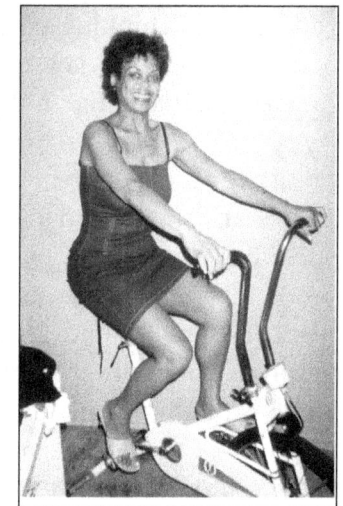
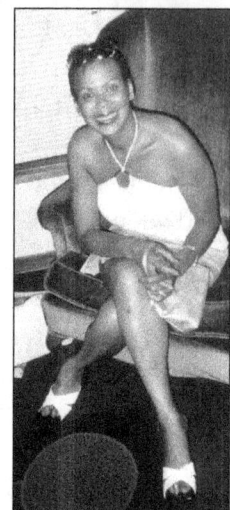
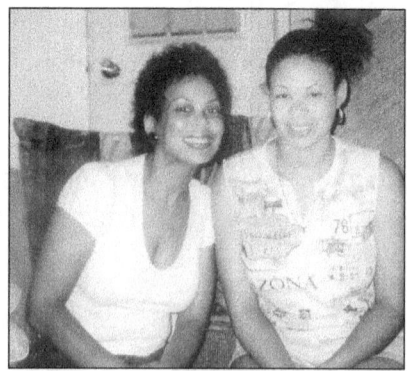

Clockwise: Me (center) during a visit to Detroit with my daughter Nicole (left), my mother-in-law Doris Dearring (seated), her daughters, Tricia, Deborah and Yvette; Me during my illness keeping a smile on my face through it all; my daughter Nicole and me.

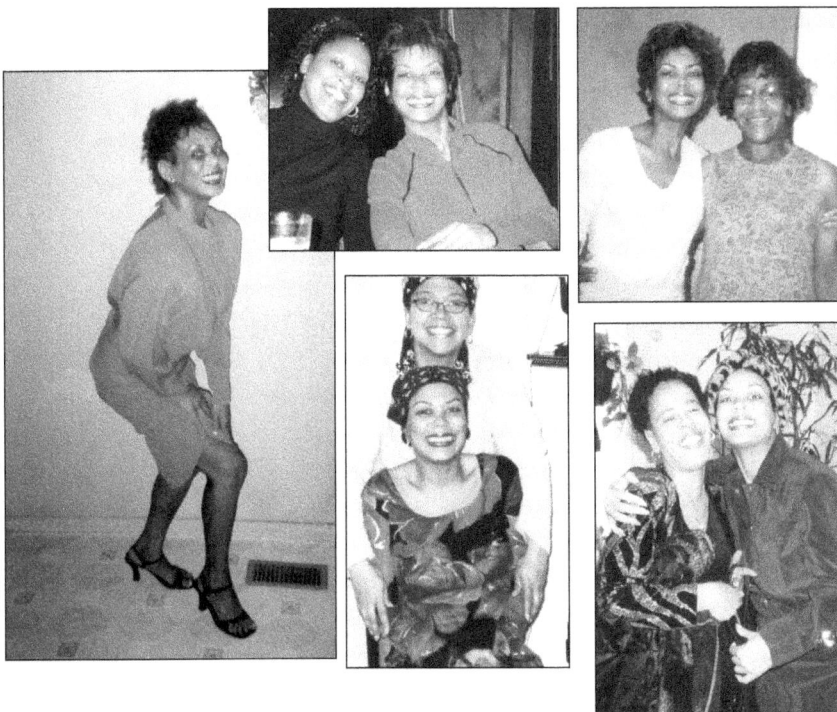

> 08/19/07
>
> Dot,
> You are truly blessed and one of God's most beautiful creations. Your loving, caring, tender and compassionate spirit has always shown in your eyes, and in your smile. You've had a hard and challenging fight, never giving up, and held on and kept the faith. You are still here, and getting stronger. August 19th is very special. Hang on to that, since it has a deeper meaning now. Another birthday is TRULY A GIFT FROM GOD. You earned it, you deserve it, and He wanted you to have it. Darlin. Much love and many blessings, Mother Judi Father Vel said Ditto 😊

Clockwise: My friend Mary Cusic as we celebrated her birthday during my illness; Mrs. Doris Dearring was a big supporter during my illness in 2001; My friend, Jeanette Payne and me during her birthday celebration; My friend, Michelle Franklin stood by me and took care of me in her home after I left the hospital in 2001; me showing my skinny legs...and my smile; a note from Mother-Judi Jones that kept me motivated as I awaited my transplant.

Chapter 6

WHO CAN FIND A VIRTUOUS WOMAN?

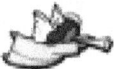

For her price is far above rubies

In 2004, my girls Esther Harden, Vee Williams, and Katie Barnes we all planned after work to go celebrate my forty-seventh birthday at Captain Luey's. Oh boy, did we have a marvelous time; never will forget dear friends. God still kept me here with a smile!

Not long after my grandsons Juan Warren II and Joshua Mann asked, "Why are you itching grandmother?"

My response, "The doctors stated that I have a rare illness, but truly I am healed in Jesus name."

Juan reply, "That is real good grandmother. We love you and don't mind giving you a helping hand to scratch that itch whenever you need us, but this is hard work."

I replied, "Believe me, this too will pass. It is only temporary; this is part of my journey."

My two grandsons looked at each other somewhat silly, not really understanding what I was trying to explain to them.

Juan said, "Grandmother, you don't look like you sick, because you always happy with a smile."

"Yes, I know," I told him. "It is my spiritual-man make-up that makes my outward appearance shine and look good. That way when people look at me they will not be able to see my pain from the inside out."

Joshua said, "Grandmother you look like cat woman." He was simply saying, I look like Halle Berry the most gorgeous movie star in Hollywood. "Only in my dreams," I laughed while they both smiled. Move over Halle Berry, I got this!

My granddaughter, Jasmine Warren also stepped up to the plate. With Jasmine being a girl, we would go to the bedroom where I could lay down while she applied ointment all over my body. My mother and niece, Anquette would also rub ointment on me in the morning and evening. The ointment was a prescription from the pharmacy in Ann Arbor, because everything I tried over the counter from the grocery stores just didn't work.

> *Be of good courage, and he shall strengthen*
> *your heart, all ye that in the Lord.*
> Psalm 31:24

It felt so good when I had someone rub the ointment on my skin to ease some of the pain of itching. I was so thankful for my beautiful grandchildren that have been there with me, especially when I need an extra hand to get that last itch! While I was waiting patiently on God for my liver, I had thoughts of suicide. "Depression must flee! I still trust you Lord," I would say to myself.

I had to stay positive and not focus on my circumstances. The one most important thing I had to remind myself was to continue trusting in God and keep my focus on Him, not my circumstances. I would listen to gospel music and the Bible on tape to speak to my body with scriptures on healing and prayer so I could keep my spiritual man fed. I sing a song called, "Yes, Jesus Loves Me." Another song I would sing was, "Oh, how I love Jesus." I learned both of these songs from my grandmothers, and in Sunday school.

There were times I felt down but bounce right back to being happy. I told myself that I wasn't going to let the devil steal my joy or let my emotions get the best of me. Repeatedly, I applied God's word in my heart with inspiration and words of encouragement to my spirit so I didn't have to mediate on the negative, but focus on God's miracle.

After four years of illness, I was still learning how to adjust and shift my physical body from my normal routine to a new lifestyle. Of course, I was not happy with it, but I had no choice or control, and had to go with the flow. The truth is, I was trying to sustain my mental state of mind by fighting the spiritual battle with Satan. God kept me in my right mind to fight the good fight of faith (I Timothy 6:12).

In the warm, hot summer month of June, my uncle, Elder Joseph C. Mann, had an eightieth birthday celebration at Ryan's Restaurant in Battle Creek. My wonderful and loving cousins, Dr. Janice Holmes and her loving husband Reverend Ben Holmes, Elder Edmon and his lovely wife, Mary Mann, and Hertis Mann pitched in together to give their dad a surprise party. My dad and I were invited to celebrate his brother's special day.

I had to make myself attend because I didn't know how much longer my devoted and lovable uncle would be with us. No matter, how I was feeling, I pressed my way to the surprise celebration with my two lovely grandchildren, Jasmine and Juan. It was good to see family, friends and his grandchildren. It meant so much to my uncle Joseph to see me. Everyone had a good time eating, talking, and taking photos. I was so grateful to have had that chance to spend time with my only living uncle.

As I struggle to press my way to church, Bishop Hugh D. Smith, Jr. and his wife, Letha Smith would always pray for me. From the first day, he heard about my illness he would continually call me up to the altar to pray and lay hands on me. The Bishop had always reminded me, "We are expecting a miracle from God, Dot. You're already healed, so walk in your healing and keep the faith in Jesus' Name."

His anointed wife would never let me leave the church without laying her healing hands located upon my stomach and pray for me. In addition, pastors Malcomb Crawford, Robert Willis, and Terris Todd, deacons Larry Henry, Tommy Kirk, Ben Gray, and other brothers of the Men's Ministries were praying for me.

Whenever I was able to arrive at Emmanuel Covenant Church International, there was Pastor Willis greeting me right at the front door as soon as I enter the church. Then, he and the other brothers would gather into the sanctuary and circle around me. We prepared to worship and pray to heaven for a miracle; doing this continually throughout my illness from day one, until it happen. I truly appreciate them for being obedient to the spirit and never quitting their prayers for me. And it didn't stop there. I also had Ethel and Keith Fitzpatrick pray for me before I would exit from the church.

One day Ethel and I were discussing why we couldn't understand why some Christians do not allow someone to pray for them when they are sick. My opinion was that Satan put it in their mind to keep it a secret from other Christians or the world so no one would be able to pray or lay hands on the individual that is going "through." Prayer is the only answer to life's situations.

My uncle passed away before his 81st birthday on April 14, 2005. Even though he is no longer with us, I believe deep down in his heart, he knew that God had already done a miracle by healing me with a new liver. This was the one thing he did not get a chance to see the blessing of the manifestation right here on earth.

Waiting for a liver transplant was not the only thing God had waiting. Even before I learned of my disease, I had no desire of a true love relationship. I have been married before and was now a divorcée. I had told myself I wouldn't get married again, because marriage is supposed to last forever (I suppose that is what Keith Sweat said in his song, "Make it Last Forever"). I guess some marriages are not meant for everyone to make it last forever. Never did I think it would ever happen to me.

When I did date, I would go to dinner, a movie, have a good time, or a friendly conversation. I didn't want any more heartbroken relationships. That is when I knew it was time to go back to my first love, Jesus. When I least expected it, spiritual love happened.

One day while I was at the store, I recognized someone who had once visited my church many years ago. His twin sister was a member and I had known her for years. That day he was leaving the store, he didn't look very happy. I passed him with my joyful smile. He stopped and approached me, reminding me that I knew his twin sister.

We began a conversation and I soon learned that he was going through a painful divorce, and was still hurt. My heart went out to him and being the congenial person I am, I wanted to say something to lift his spirits.

When he asked if I had remarried?

"No, I been waiting for you," I said laughing.

"Yeah, right," he said blushing.

I was ill, but was not thinking about my condition... can a girl has some fun? We exchanged phone numbers and a friendly hug before we both went our way. Battle Creek is a small town, but there are times when you have no idea how often you will cross paths with someone. After about three months, he called me. He said he had lost my number and had surprisingly gotten it from one of his friend. He admitted that when we met he was seeing someone. However, with that relationship over and he wanted to connect with me. He said he admired my heart, and wanted to get to know me better.

As time passed, we talked about how important it was to have God at the center of it all—something that wasn't there in my first marriage. My last marriage came filled with challenges from alcohol and substance abuse. The shame and embarrassment felt by the both of us in our last relationships led to us being cautious and vowed never to marry again. Calvin said he could relate.

Although we would talk for hours, I didn't want to tell Calvin about my illness. I was in the early stage of my liver disease and unless you notice my itching, little else about me said I was sick. I thanked God that I was not still suffering emotionally from the divorce. I had put up walls when men approached me for a long time. I knew there were still some good men in the world; I just had not come across meeting the right one yet. This time I will allow the Lord to choose him, because my choice in men has been unequally yoked.

When a sista' goes through an intimate relationship she pours her heart and soul out to a man, often all that is left is a broken heart and pain. It is very difficult to build up the walls of love and trust in any man. I made many mistakes when it came to worldly love because Jesus' love was not in it.

But God had to heal my heart just as I was dealing with my illness. It was time to open my heart and forgive – by moving forward - getting rid of all bitterness and hatred had to flee in Jesus' name. I had to move on and let go, and be able to love with compassion and be happy with myself spiritually. I recognized God's divine love whenever I was around my father and stepmother.

At first, I did not understand why my parents divorced. I couldn't help but see how good my dad and stepmother were made for one another. Together they were growing spiritually, prosperity, and working together in many ways. By watching them, I realized the importance of being "equally yoked" spiritually and it does plays an important role in life.

After about six months, I decided to invite Calvin to my home. By then, I had explained my diagnosis of cirrhosis of the liver, but not the itching. He had heard–like many people–that cirrhosis came from liver deterioration after alcohol abuse. He was surprise to learn that all I had been experiencing over the years dispelled that myth. Soon after, I had to share of my intense itching fits, just so he would be aware. After an initial greeting, hug and tour of my home, he seemed impressed. I tried so hard not to itch, but the feeling was becoming more than I could hide. I explained it to him and began to scratch!

"I suppose you can leave if you like too," I said to him, feeling he would not want to be around someone who did this all day.

"I'm your friend, I'm here for you," he said smiling. "That's what a real man, a Godly man is here on earth for. Even after looking at you, I would have never even thought you was sick or had a condition, if you hadn't told me." Therefore, he decided to stay and pray for me.

His words meant more than I could have imagined. Our friendship continued, mostly by phone. I shared information about my liver transplant and how I hung on to the words of my uncle Joseph who always said, "You're healed in Jesus name; keep speaking it to your body every day, Dottie May."

Therefore I say unto to you, What things so ever ye desire, when ye pray believe that ye receive them and ye shall them.
Mark 11:24

One day while talking to Calvin on the phone, I was not feeling my best. I was getting worse and forgetful, but still holding on to God's Word. There were times Calvin wanted to see me, but I was not in any condition in seeing anyone. I only had time to be intimate with God.

In August, I left Battle Creek to ride with my dad and Hertis Mann to Atlanta, Georgia to see my gorgeous Edith Harvey and family. I also want to visit my sweet and beautiful Aunt Mary (who was the only girl living siblings on my dad's side of the family) and other loving relatives in Georgia.

Calvin had phoned me to let me know that his divorce has been final and if we could be more than friends?

I said, "I don't understand? I am in no condition to have a relationship with anyone right now. What is it that you want? Why don't you get someone that is healthy and beautiful?"

"All I want is you, and I don't want anyone else," he said.

I was speechless and impressed. I asked Calvin to let me spend time with my relatives and think about it. "Right now I need no confusion, no drama or stress from no one. I only need to focus on Jesus. What do I have to offer you?"

"Only your heart," he answered.

2006

Over the years, in dealing with the physical ailments that come with liver disease, I have used a variety of antidepressant medications such as Zoloft. While I stay encouraged through the word of God, there were just some things I could not control some through prayer. I often had to lay in bed all day because of lack of energy.

I became more and more frustrated with life. Sometimes I found it very hard to tolerate noise. Besides that, I had a lack of appetite in addition to dealing with everything else that was going on. The sores constantly appeared on my body. Oh Lord, what else more could happen?

As I still smiled for everyone who came around me. I had become more forgetful, had trouble sleeping, and feelings of frustration. The liver issues with the body's ability to process vitamin D and calcium (both needed for strong bones) to keep from making my bones brittle and weak. The doctor prescribed Actonel to deal with the bone loss or to prevent osteoporosis. This disease was taking a toll on me physically and mentally.

There were times I felt at my lowest. I wondered what was going to happen, and when it was going to end. Even my teeth started to bother because of the lack of vitamins in my body. Regardless of how much calcium or vitamins I swallowed on a daily basis, nothing I did could save some of my teeth pearly whites. Gradually, through my journey I had to schedule many dentists' appointments to help save some of my teeth.

What kind of mountains or obstacles do you have in your life right now? Obey, Jesus and his commandments that mountain of pain, cancer, whatever afflicts your body be healed. Do not listen to your body. Listen to Jesus! That's what I had to do. It seemed like the constant itching and sores on my skin were arising daily. Some were so small that I thought they were pimples. Between that and the pain, I was on the verge of depression, but I would stop that thinking immediately and prayed.

And Jesus answering saith unto them, have faith in God. For verily I say unto you, That whosoever shall say unto this mountain, Be thou removed, and be thou cast into the sea; and shall not doubt in his heart, but shall believe that those things which he saith shall come to pass; he shall have whatsoever he saith.
Mark 11:22-23

There were things I wanted to do, but I felt helpless and worthless when I couldn't do the simple things to take care of myself. Sometimes my moods would lead to thoughts that no one cared, if I lived or died. Even suicidal thoughts tried to defeat me, but I quickly realized that it was a stupid idea! There is no option to quit! I knew, in the back of my mind, that none of those negative thoughts was true. I had to believe in my heart, JESUS loves me and that is all that matters.

I had to keep speaking to my spirit with scriptures like, "I can do all things through Christ which strengthen me" (Philippians 4:13). No matter what came my way, I was still alive, living, loving and enjoying the spiritual good life of Jesus Christ. The best was yet to come; the Lord would always make a way out of no way...only on His own time.

May 2006

As my dad and I continued driving to Chicago for follow-up tests, I knew it was the Christ in him that gave him energy, strength and love to keep going for me. He never complained. Because Chicago time was an hour behind Michigan time, the appointments always seemed to take longer. Sometimes we wouldn't get back to Battle Creek until after 11 p.m.

It was at those times that I felt I should be taking care of him. I had been so independent my whole life. Having him, families, friends and church members whenever I needed them was a blessing. He was getting up in age and he was taking care of me. God bless my daddy.

I know my dad's crown is waiting next to mine in heaven. Sometime I would wish upon a star that if I had a magic wand to take all my pain and sickness away so I could go on living like an ordinary, normal people without my dad, or anyone taking care of me anyway.

After my illness had been revealed throughout the community, the Holy Spirit put it in me not to be shameful or discouraged about myself. I was never to hide, but to be a witness and a "chosen vessel" for the Lord, and to let the world know that Jesus lives in me.

> *But ye are a chosen generation, a royal priesthood, an holy nation, a peculiar people; that ye should shew forth the praises of him who hath called you out of darkness into his marvelous light: Which in time past were not a people, but are now the people of God: which had not obtained mercy, but now have obtained mercy.*
> I Peter 2:9-10

I knew then that nonbelievers and Christians would look at me to see how I was handling my situation. I knew that when God delivered me from my sickness, the world would know that He is a healer and still does miracles! Thank you God, that no one can see the sores in my head, except for my lovely hairdresser, Patricia Prince.

Sometime listening to motivational messages just were not enough. When the opportunity came to see Rev. Peter Popoff in Detroit, my sista' girl, Meria, drove Calvin and I to see the pastor who was known for healing beside Benny Hinn. I wanted to be part of it. The hotel banquet room was filled with people waiting to experience this healing. Everyone in the room was asked to hold someone hand next to them and pray.

When I reached for the hand of the girl next to me, she said in disgust, "You have Lupus all over your body. It's a disease, please don't touch me." I was hurt and turned to Calvin who was upset about the comment. After that, the mood didn't seem welcoming, and we left for home.

Whenever the immune system gets low my body couldn't fight off the germs or bacteria. The results could be:

1) Shingles would affect my body and spread intensely, leading to itching all over my back with burning pain. At times, I couldn't wear clothes unless they were cotton.

2) Various skin rashes would appear on my stomach and back.

3) Osteoporosis would begin. Tests on my hipbone showed I was on the brink of other metabolic bone diseases that could appear at the usual time. The swelling from the fluid build-up in my legs and ankles (called Edema) were in severe pain. At times, I could hardly walk or stand up more than three days. It would go away, and then without notice, it happens again.

As I awaited the approval from the hospital to receive a new liver, I prayed, "Come on my new liver I need you, so I shall live for my purposes. I have not finished the course of my journey. I will continually wait patiently and hold on a little bit longer. A change is coming!"

I kept belief in God's word no matter what and how bad or good the circumstance looked. I had to look over ignorant people, what they thought or said about me, and pray for them. At times like these, I would say to myself, "I will trust in you Lord!"

Symptoms in liver disease:

- Abnormal yellow discoloration of the skin and eyes. This is called Jaundice often the first sometimes the only sign of liver disease
- Dark urine
- Gray, yellow or light-colored stools
- Nausea, vomiting and/or loss of appetite
- Vomiting of blood, bloody or black stools. Intestinal bleeding can occur with diseases obstruct blood flow through the liver. The bleeding may result in blood or bloody stools
- Abdominal swelling. Liver disease may cause ascites, an ac cumulation of abdominal cavity
- Prolonged, generalized itching
- Unusual change of weight
- Abdominal pain
- Sleep disturbances, mental confusion, and coma are present in severe live result from an accumulation of toxic substances in the body
- Fatigue or loss of stamina
- Loss of sexual drive or performance

And we know that all things work together for good to them that love the Lord and are the called according to the will of God.

Romans 8:28

Chapter 7

STORY OF JOB

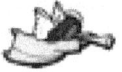

Why do people suffer? I never understood the true meaning of, suffering until I had to go through my own experiences of long-suffering. This experience is something I would not wish on my worst enemies.

One Sunday morning, after church service I humbly walked over to talk to my Bishop. I explain to him how difficult the past five years has been with the sores, lack of sleep and constant itching. Truly, I wasn't complaining. He understood my frustrations and quickly lay hands (of prayer) on me and keep him up-to-date about what is going on with my condition.

As our Shepherd, he is dearly concerned when someone going through a difficult time because he knows each one of his sheep spiritual personally. He knows we all have to face the storms of life, and go through trials and tribulation. He then told me about the man in the Bible, *Job* and that I should read that chapter to see the similarities in our stories.

In the King James translation of *Job*, the story is set during the time of the Patriarchs (about 2000-1800 B.C.). Satan attacked Job's health in Job 2:1-10. In the *Spirit-Filled Life Bible for Students* it reads: *Satan brings sickness and disease to Job* (Job 2:4-8).

It is interesting to note that Satan attacked Job's physical health. The Bible teaches us that sickness is not always the result of germs, viruses, infections, chemicals, or pollution. Sometime sickness is a specific attack from demonic powers and Satan. In the New Testament, we see that when Jesus Christ healed people there was always a close relationship between physical healing and the casting out of demons *(Matthew 10:1, 7- 8; 12:22-29).*

At the end of Job's journey, many people talked about his sufferings, but the fact is that God did not leave Job in a state of poverty, sickness, and suffering. The Lord gave him twice as much as had before. God not only taught Job a valuable lesson from which we all can learn, but also returned him to a place of blessing and joy.

> *And these things we write unto you, that your joy may be full.*
> *This is the message, which we have heard of HIM, and declare unto you, that God is light, and in HIM is no darkness at all.*
> *If we say that we have fellowship with HIM, and walk darkness, we lie, and do not have truth; But if we walk in the light, as he is in the light, we have fellowship one with another, and the blood of Jesus Christ his Son cleans us from all sin.*
> (John 1:4-7)

The way of the blessing is to walk in the blessing! It was time to reveal my blessing with my name on it. I, like Job, suffered sores from the top of my head to the bottom of my foot. When Satan attacked my life, he was trying to make me believe that I was going to lose my mind and lose my home. I had no purpose, no dreams, or no desire to live. He tried to steal my joy and make me doubt my faith.

> *So Satan answered the Lord and said, "Skin for skin! Yes, all that a man has he will give for his life. But stretch out your hand now, and touch his bone and his flesh, and he will surely curse you to your face!"*
>
> *And the Lord said to Satan,*
> *"Behold, he is in your hand, but spare his life."*
>
> *So Satan went out from the presence of the Lord, and struck Job with painful boils from the sole of his foot to the crown of his head. And he took for himself a potsherd with which to scrape himself while he sat in the midst of the ashes. Then his wife said to him, "Do you still hold fast to your integrity? Curse God and die!"*
>
> *But he said to her, "You speak as one of the foolish women speaks. Shall we indeed accept well from God, and shall we not accept adversity?" In all this Job did not sin with his lips.*
> (Job 2:4-9)

At first, I did not understand why Bishop asked me to read *Job*. Now, I know. I could relate to some of the experiences *Job* had to go through. That's amazing! If you ever want to question anything in life, read the Bible. It will tell you everything you need to know in today's life issues. For me, the story of Job relates to my situation of the sores. I learned to be obedience to the spirit, fear God, and hate Satan.

Then I asked a question, "Why, me Lord?"

God spoke to my spirit, "Why not you, daughter? Who are you? You are no different than anybody else."

"Why, not my sister and brother?" I asked.

"Well, because I chose you to represent me so you can show the world your faith that I, God, is *real*, and miracles do happen if people believe it or not, it comes through me. As far as your other sibling, they are not saved and I knew they wouldn't be able to stand the test of faith in my name."

I felt ashamed. I fell down on my knees to bow down and worship the King. I asked the Lord for forgiveness, and said I would never ever question God again!

Every day was a struggle when it was time to do any routine work. I was slow to anger and never complained about the little things that I didn't have control of, for one thing life is too precious and too short. I was thankful for every day I had a job and I was alive. When my health couldn't hold up any longer and my liver was not functioning properly like a regular liver, I had to remind myself to stand and wait on God to get my liver. I refused to give up!

My expectation and determination is to get what belongs to me and I am not going to let Satan or anyone stand in my way. The one thing I did learn in all of this, if you're *not* connected to God, and have good health and no faith, how could you truly enjoy a good life? You are only going through the motions of pretending to be living, but truly is it living?

I cannot image anyone living a good life without Christ. Some unbelievers do it every day; living in the world acting happy, but sad on the inside. In reality, they may be lost and are just going through the motions in *sin*, but there is no Jesus living inside of them.

The one important thing that was taught by my parents and grandmother, "To treat and respect everyone the way you would want to be treated; which is to be kind." This is something that this generation does not seem to have, which means, "Be kind to others and *blessing* will come back to you."

At the time when I was weak, vulnerable and confused and it seemed that even the physicians in Michigan couldn't do anything further to help me. The only person I could turn to in the midnight hour was my heavenly father. Even with my short-term memory, and trouble concentrating, and homicidal suicide thoughts, I knew that one day when it is all over I could tell the world that God loves me.

Toward the end, I began to keep a journal. I was told by the Holy Spirit, to write this story to share with others. (I recalled when mother Cherrie Williams had spoken to me about keeping a journal during my illness. Now, I learned if you ever want to tell a story keep a journal.)

Behold, we count them happy, which endure, Ye have heard of the patience of Job, and have seen the end of the Lord: that the Lord is very pitiful, and of tender mercy.
James 5:11

No weapon that is formed against thee shall prosper; and every tongue that shall rise against thee in judgement thou shalt condemn.

Isaiah 54:17

Chapter 8

YOU GOT TO PUT A RING ON IT!

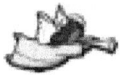

In June, Calvin and I discussed planning a vacation to Disney World to celebrate my 50th Birthday (August 19). Two weeks before my birthday he asked me to marry him and I said, No. He had proposed to me before, but I had said, "If you want to marry me, you will have to put a ring on it, then my answer will be, Yes!" So he did. He had bought me a gorgeous diamond ring from Zale's Jewelry.

At first, I thought Calvin wanted to marry me because I was sick. Maybe he was just feeling sorry for me or wanted to show me some happiness during my last days on earth. I did not know what to think.

"First, I get my liver, and then I marry you. It might be a long wait," I said.

Calvin replied, "I will wait."

"When we do get married, I am going to walk down the aisle with my handsome dad. You will be standing there with a twinkle of love in your eyes looking at your queen coming down the aisle….looking at her sexy King." And that's what we did…wait.

My birthday was a lovely, bright, sunny, and hot day to be alive. There is something about birthdays—it is a joyful blessing to see another birthday. Five years passed, and I don't' think anyone expected me to still be alive. But I was. And I was smiling, and happy that I was turning 50, and looking fabulous! My sister Ola, and my daughter Nicole, planned a surprise birthday party for me.

On that beautiful morning, I had appointment to go to my hairdresser Pattie Prince. My sister and daughter had phoned me to see what I had planned for that day. My fiancé had to work and planned to take me out that weekend. Earlier that morning his sister Meria wanted to take me out to dinner. Time was quickly passing, and I was running behind schedule. Meria was on her way to pick me up about 5 p.m. to go to dinner.

After I left the hairdresser, I was not feeling my best. But once again, I pressed my way to getting dressed; I was not going to have anything spoil my birthday. There were many dearest friends and families calling to wish me happy birthday. She took me to the clubhouse off Dickman Road where guests were waiting quietly inside. My daughter came to the car to help me up the stairs because I was feeling a little tired.

As I enter the door I heard, "Surprise!"

There I saw my parents, stepmother Ethel, sister Ola and her husband, Kathy Mabry, Michael Edwards, Linda Cooper, her mother, Mrs. Hughes, my grandchildren, Jasmine, Juan, Joshua, and many more wonderful friends. The evening was engaging and delightful with love. What a bash!

✲✲✲

Ever since I was a child, I wanted to see Mickey and Minnie Mouse. Neither Calvin nor I had ever been to Florida, so we decide to go to Disney World in Orlando to celebrate both of our birthdays that were in August.

Once we arrived, a large painful rash appeared across my stomach. There nothing I could do about it, but pray. The Shingles were attacking my immune system. Here I go again! The itching and Shingles had come together to make my trip unpleasant. But, I wasn't going to allow anything to spoil our romantic vacation in Florida. The trip turned out to be so lovely. It was a special time for the two of us, and an awesome birthday gift to remember for the rest of our lives.

One day while in Florida, I could see that there were times when Calvin wanted to speak his mind or lash out at those people who stared or pointed at me. Some people were whispering aloud while making fun of the spots on my body. I will never forget the little boy who pointed his finger at me and began to laugh at my spots. His mother smacked him right in the mouth. She told him not to ever do that again because it was rude. In the back of my mind, I wanted to praise her for teaching her child respect and not to point or talk about an individual's appearance. I wish more mothers were more like her. It made me smiled. Other than that, Calvin and I had a marvelous time. It was the perfect time to get away. Maybe one day we will return to Disney World when I am healthy.

The dermatologist in Chicago had carefully diagnosed the spots on my skin as "Lichen Planus." They will not disappear until I had a liver transplant. Until then, I would have to deal with the pain, bruises, and itching that kept appearing on my skin. I had an ointment to help ease some of the pain, but it didn't work. I learned to block out the vision and try not to focus on those ugly spots.

Lichen Plamus is a common skin disease; it is an inflammatory condition that can affect your skin and mucous membranes. On the skin, lichen planus usually appears as purplish, often itchy, flat-topped bumps on the arm or legs. It is a chronic rash characterized by scaly skin plaques.

I tried hard not to dwell or think on negative thoughts, or focus on the swelling in my legs and ankles that could sometimes make it difficult to walk. With the change in my skin texture and various skin rashes, I tried to overlook foolish people when they saw something awful upon my legs and arms. At times, I felt like running to hide and never show myself again. But the Holy Spirit would not allow me too.

November 2006

I finally had to come to conclusion about my situation and my health. I would have wear a bandana to cover my thinning hair and the bald spots where large sores had appeared. There were times I tried not to focus on my outward appearance as long as I had my smile!

One day, I spoke with my supervisors Fred Elizondo and Jeff VandenBoss about how I had prayed about my circumstances at work. It became more exhausting and harder to perform my duties as an employee. It was time to leave my job and focus on God's purposes.

After working five years on the job with this illness, I submitted my paperwork to the Office Personnel Management at the Federal Center regarding my retirement disability. I was so grateful and appreciative of my supervisors for their generous time, expertise, and help during my time of need. Their was no way I could have done it alone. I love them both dearly, in Jesus' name.

As we waited to hear response back from the personnel office, I talked to Bishop, my dad, and Calvin as I prayed about it. I knew deep in my spirit and heart, it was time to remove myself from my job by closing this chapter of my life.

Due to the progression of my disease, I was suffering from other complications, which were preventing me from working a full-time job or on a part-time basis. When is God's miracle going to happen in my life? I begin to feel speechless; not knowing the day or hour when it will take place...only God knows. I told myself, "I will trust Him and His plans for me. I believe whole-heartedly it is time to retire from the Federal Center."

November 13, 2006

My doctor suggested a procedure called Plasmapheresis, that could get my number counts higher on the transplant list. My enzymes were very low. It seemed like we had tried everything in the doctor's medial book to get rid of this itching. At this point in my life I would tried anything, so I did. Because I was under care for secondary to Primary Biliary Cirrhosis (PBC) and I was currently on the Liver Transplant waiting list. Amen! By needing this device, it would show the severity of my condition and the immediate need for a liver.

Plasmapheresis is a method of removing blood plasma from the body by withdrawing blood, separating it into plasma and cells, and transfusing the cells back into the bloodstream. In sick people, plasma can contain antibodies that attack the immune system. A machine removes the affected plasma and replaces it with good plasma, or a plasma substitute. This is also known as plasma exchange. During Plasmapheresis, blood is removed from the body and passed through a machine that separates blood cells.

It is perform specially to remove antibodies in treating autoimmune conditions. Plasmapheresis is a blood purification procedure used to treat several autoimmune diseases. It is also known as therapeutic plasma exchange. Replacement or returned plasma flows in to the body through a second tube that is place in the arm or foot. A patient can need as many as five treatments per week. Plasmapheresis is defined as the removal…diseases of unknown cause–William ME

December 2006

In the meantime, I did what I had to do to stop the itching. All I want is to get well. Therefore, for next six weeks I did the blood plasma. I can never be disappointed in my heavenly father, because HE is the one that is keeping me here. God has been good to me. Even when I had not been good to myself, God was all I had.

God understood everything I was going through in the midst of my suffering—even though at times I could not function, I knew angels were looking out for me. I hereby take authority, "Sickness, take your hands off my body!" Satan tried to continue to make me think negative thoughts and to bring harm to myself, but I continued to pray daily, be patience and quiet.

I thought about when I got my breakthrough, and being an overcomer to let people know who God is. Even Satan knew I had the victory in Jesus' name. I hoped and prayed that the people around me saw His goodness, hope, and faith, no matter how bad it may have seemed. I was in a spiritual fight and had to use scriptures as my weapon.

It is better to trust in the Lord than to put confidence in man.
Psalm 118:8

> *Death and life are in the power of the tongue;*
> *and they that love shall eat the fruit thereof.*
> Proverbs 18:21

I had to hold on, in good times or bad. I keep on worship and praising His name. Mother Rosie, Darlene Morris and Antoinette Hardeman gave me wisdom during my storm.

Mother Rosie stated, "When taking medicine, mix faith with it by saying, 'I believe, I receive my healing in Jesus Name.' You must know that most medicine will help hold down the symptoms while you are applying God's principles concerning healing and health."

She also stated that some Christians do not believe in seeing a doctor, but trust in the Lord to heal them. What some of those thinkers don't understand is that God puts doctors here on earth to help heal. It is also true that doctors don't always understand the diagnosis they give. That is why a second evaluation from other physicians is important. If you believe God will heal, apply faith daily and God will do the rest.

Darlene and Antoinette continue to ask me to speak scriptures out loudly on healing. Listen to Bishop Smith and Creflo Dollar's recorded messages on CD's daily. My dad said, "Play your gospel music through the night, singing hymns songs (my favorite song "Oh how I love Jesus), especially in the midnight hour." I had to learn not to feel sorry about my illness and what I had to go through, but to believe and speak with a positive attitude.

Mother Cherrie Williams allowed me to continue listening to her Bible scriptures on CD to stay encourage, because it was very difficult for me to focus while reading the Bible and itching. I worked to ease my spiritual body, but there was never peace from the itching of my physical body. The devil is steady trying to get inside my head bring craziness, negative, depression and suicidal thoughts as I lay in bed.

"I have the authority to command wisdom, I am a happy person, and I shall live and not die," I said it repeatedly to my spiritual man.

There's Something Behind That Smile

Now faith is the substance of things hoped for,
the evidence of things not seen.
Hebrew 11:1

But as for you, ye thought evil against me; but God meant it unto
good, to bring to pass, as it is this day, to save much people alive.
Genesis 50:20

Jesus said unto him, "If thou canst believe, all things
are possible to him that to believeth.
Mark 9:23

I delight to do thy will, O my God: yea, thy law is within my heart.
Psalm 40:8

Jesus answered, Verily, verily, I say unto thee, Except a man
be born of water and of the Spirit, he cannot enter
into the kingdom of God that is born of flesh is flesh:
and that which is born of the Spirit is spirit.
John 3:5-6

On January 2007, I received a letter from the Office of Personnel, which read: "...*this letter is to inform you that your application for disability retirement under Civil Service Retirement System has been approved.*"

I was excited and jumped up for joy right there at my desk. I quietly shout out to heaven in my spirit, "Thank you, thank you dear Lord." I gave out a loud shout when it came to Jesus' name, because it was something about that named, Jesus. It is something I'm not ashamed to say, I know Him.

I move swiftly towards the rest room where I shouted and rejoiced loudly. At this point, I did not care who heard me. "Hallelujah, I'm out of here!" I said.

There will be people on the job I would miss dearly, but in my spirit, I knew it was time to move on. I knew I had to call it quits! I was retiring after more than twenty-six years of working there.

I tried hard not to show tears. The people I had worked with had been so nice and care about me, and I made sure to let them know how much I really appreciate them being important part of my life. Everyone waved and blew kisses as I departed. "Thank you all for so much love, KAEA!"

Craig, one of my coworkers, helped me carry my boxes to the car. It was very, very hard to leave as I cried my way from the building to my car. I will never forget the ones who were always there for me. Some had blessed me with delightful cards, bringing food to my home, gave me personal leave and donations. I was no longer a civilian employee at the Battle Creek Federal Center, but a retired one who would receive disability benefits. When I looked back on my life, I was truly blessed to have an amazing job at the Federal Center as a family that will always be in my heart.

***

In the month of January 2007, I had to return to Northwestern Memorial Hospital for follow-up blood work and tests. My condition seemed to have gotten worse than before–especially the itching. The doctors and I decided once again to submit another letter to the board of hospital for a liver transplant. This would be our third time. I was on the bottom of the waiting list because doctors didn't seemed to see me as a very sick person. (Anyone who knew me would thought the same as if I had lost a lot of weight.)

On this particular Sunday morning at church, Bishop called me to come up in front of the congregation to the altar. He began to pray for me, put blessing oil on my head, and lay his anointed hands upon my stomach. God was doing a spiritual operation at that moment, where the heavenly doors opened up. One day it will happen; the manifestation of the operation will take place right here on earth.

On January 23, 2007, I received a letter from the Defense Logistics Information Service at Hart-Dole-Inouye Federal Center in Battle Creek.

Dear Ms. Dearring:

I want to take this opportunity to thank you for your service to the U.S. Government over the past 26-plus years. I hope you have improved health and are able to enjoy your retirement.

Sincerely, John Fitzgerald, Commander

February 2007

Two weeks after I left, my supervisor Fred Elizondo, and Janet Bash, planned a retirement party for me. This would give me the opportunity to go back and see some of the other people I didn't get a chance to say goodbye to earlier. My future sister-in-law Meria Wyrick, came along. The room was exquisite, colorfully decorated with balloons, trays of assorted food beautifully laid out and deliciously tasty. Everyone who attended had something nice to say about me. I felt love in the atmosphere and I wasn't going to hold back the tears.

April 2007

I received a letter from the hospital saying that I was approved for a liver transplant! During Wednesday night Bible study, I couldn't wait to tell Bishop Smith that I was place at the top of the list to receive a liver. When he heard the good news, he smiled. I told several other leaders and a few more church members the good news. Going to Bible study allowed me to be fed spiritually. It was something I had continued to do throughout my illness. Through it all, I had continued to sing praises to God, worship and pay my tithes.

Bishop Smith asked, "Have they called you yet?"

I would say, "No, not yet!"

"The call is coming," he said.

All I could do was smile. Still, at times it would be very difficult to be relaxed or not scratch around other people. I would ask the Holy Spirit to speak to me during these times. As long as I was singing praises, it took the focus off my pain and frustration. I should be very grateful where the Lord has brought me from during this difficult time in my life. I speak to my body with authority; I receive that life through God's word. I read scriptures such as:

> *Being confident of this very thing, that he which hath begun a good work in you will perform it until the day of Jesus Christ*
> Philippians 1:6

> *The thief cometh not, but for to steal, and to kill, and to destroy: I am come that they might have life, and that they might have it more abundantly.*
> John 10:10

> *It is the Spirit who gives life; the flesh profits nothing. The words that I speak to you are spirit, and they are life.*
> John 6:63

My uncle's Joseph favorite scripture is Isaiah 53:5. He told me to speak it every day aloud to my spirit. I spoke that I was healed in the name of Jesus and that my believing I would be healed. Therefore, I did. I believe and receive by faith that I am healed.

> *Heal me, O Lord, and I shall be healed; save me, and I shall be saved: for thou art my praise.*
> Jeremiah 17:14

In May, 2007, my day-to-day living was subject to change based on my illness. There was time I could not get out of bed, take a shower, and prepare meals, to take my medication or even breathe without an issue. All I could think about is getting my new liver and becoming healthy again. I knew the Lord was with me and I continued to call on him and worship in the spirit. There were many times when my physical body wanted me to throw in the towel. My heart said something different.

> *He sent his word, and healed them, and delivered them from their destructions.*
> Psalm 107:20

Aunt Violet Kelly, Doris Dearring and Dr. Janice Holmes along with many dearest friends and family would call on me daily. Every day, there were people on the prayer line to heaven on by behalf. These people included my lovely parents, fiancé, stepmother Ethel, relatives, Bishop Smith and his wife Letha, Pastors Donna Simmons, Tino Smith, Graham and his lovely wife Sandy, and church members.

It was good to know that so many people loved me. I had to learn that through my experiences of physical sickness, long-suffering and affliction. Submit yourselves therefore to God. "Resist the devil, and he will flee from you"(James 4:7). Sickness is a part of a curse of Satan, not the Lord. Christ died for our sins and it is by his stripes we are healed. Therefore, I give no place to sickness or pain. Amen

During the waiting, I learned to count my blessing and not take life lightly or for granted–especially your health. I learned to never feel sorry for myself when life doesn't go our way, just give the situation to God and pray. The only request I asked from anyone was to keep me in prayers so that I shall live and not die. I was never to doubt God in my heart. "Only to believe that those things which he saith shall come to pass; he shall have whatsoever he saith" (Mark 11:23).

I looked back to where it all began in 2001. I was helpless in the hospital at Battle Creek Health System for two weeks. I had come so far. I was still here, in Jesus' name. I remember God and I had a little chat, and I said:

Lord,

If it is your will and it's my time to die, I may not understand that, but if you do decided to take me to heaven, Lord, I will continually talk [to the Lord] so much that I will not be able to be quiet. So Lord, please think about it! And if by any chance it is your will to keep me here on earth, believe me, I will share my testimony of healing to everyone to hear around the world. They may be going through sickness and need to hear a word of encouragement. I will spread the good news in your name and give you all the highest glory because this is not about me, it is all about you.

Along with physical and emotional changes over the past years, no matter how I felt, I kept the faith! I also recalled the statement made by Joni, the registered nurse who said, "usually after five or six years a patient will see more serious complications in their condition."

> *Again I say unto you. That if two of you shall agree on Earth as touching anything they shall ask, it shall be done for them of my Father which is in heaven. For where two or three are gathered together in my name, there am I in the midst of them.*
> Matthew 18:19-20

One Wednesday night Bible study, Bishop taught a lesson on, "Believe and Receive your Faith." When I approached him, he asked, as always, "Have they called you yet?"

"No, not yet, Bishop!"

"You might as well get prepare, because the call is coming and your liver is on its way," he would confirm as we both rejoiced.

The *Spirit Filled Life Bible for Students* states, the key word in the Gospel of John is "believe." It is faith that unlocks our understanding of Scripture, and it is faith that releases the Holy Spirit's activity within our lives. If we are to walk in faith and live victoriously, we must believe in the miracles of Jesus (vv. 37, 38) and understand that the glory of God is reveal to those who believe (11:40).

Faith, like love, shows evidence through obedience. What we practice of God's Word is what bring blessing to ourselves and to others (13:17). There is absolutely no way to know God except to know Jesus, because Jesus is the only way to God; and we must choose to believe this if we are to have a relationship with HIM (14:6-7; see also Hebrew 11:6). We must believe!

> *If I do not the works of my Father, believe me not. But if I do, though ye believe not me, believe the works: that ye may know, and believe, that the Father is in me, and I in him.*
> John 10:37-38

Whenever I begin to itch, I tried to pretend to stay still. At this stage of my life, it was very difficult to wear clothing that rubbed up against my skin with the sores upon my body. I whispered softly to my spirit, "Help me Lord, not to remove my (irritating) clothing in public. I sang a song to my spirit, "Oh how I love Jesus, because He first loved me… because the Bible tells me so."

Brother Keith Fitzpatrick had stopped me at the door entrance of the church. He whispered in my ear, giving me inspirational words to my spirit and to let me know to, "receive your blessing from the Lord." He said, "You must believe in your heart, what God is getting ready to do for you. Remember, God loves you , Dot." We both smiled.

When I was leaving the church on my way home, I happened to look up at the clouds. I could feel it in my spirit that my miracle was coming soon. I smiled.

I was five years old when my grandmother told me about a man named Jesus, who died on the cross so that we could live and be healed of all transgressions of disease—that is if you can believe. I also remember both grandmothers who loved Jesus. They read Bible stories to my sisters and me. They would say, "Jesus loves all the little children of the world. He is the best thing that could ever happen to a child." Today, I can say, "I am <u>still</u> one of them."

Jesus saith unto him, I am the way, the truth, and the life: no man cometh unto the Father, but by me.
John 14:6

In June of 2007, my illness was changing rapidly. I was scheduled to see a psychiatrist Dr. TK, and my cousin, Kathy Mabry came along with me. As I was waiting to see the doctor, one of the nurses made a stupid comment pertaining to me while talking to the receptionist. She said that I wasn't going to make it. Kathy was unhappy and there was unspeakable sadness in her voice.

After the session with the doctor, Kathy slowly helped me to the car. I could see there was something bothering her. She whispered, "Dot, did you hear what the nurse had said to the receptionist about you?"

"No!"

"Good!" she said. "And thank God, you didn't hear it."

It was a good thing that the Holy Spirit didn't allow me to hear such foolishness. I was going to get what God had for me—my new liver.

Later that evening, because of the forgetfulness of memory and the confusion that was going on in my head, I was referred to Borgess Hospital in Kalamazoo, about twenty minutes from Battle Creek. After the results of the blood work earlier, it had been determined that my liver was failing and my kidneys were barely functioning.

I called my fiancé and his sister to tell them what was going on. Meria drove me to the hospital and Calvin rode along with us. Once we arrived, I wanted to go back home, but I was in no condition mentally to take care of myself. My physical body had quickly moved into secondary stage liver disease. My body was deteriorating quickly.

No one in my family had any idea about how bad of shape I was in. I had told my dad and my best girl, Esther not to say a word about me being in the hospital. I didn't want to alarm or worry any more of my family. In a wink of an eye, the shingles reappeared, attacking my immune system and turning my situation from bad to worst.

This time I had developed a deep large thick horizontal line across my back that brought pain as if a fire was burning from within my body. I couldn't lay on my back or rest comfortably. All through the night, I asked the Lord to help. I couldn't get any sleep or peace of mind and the itching and scratching continued. I had moved from one end of the room, praising and worshipping to the other end of the room. It was all I had at this point, through this difficult time. I needed peace in mind in my soul and body.

At that moment, I was thinking about my mother's affection and my dad's strength. I wish they both had been here by my side if only to give a hug and to hold my hand. But I had to remind myself, God is right here with me and He will not forsake me; God loves me and had been by my side from the beginning.

Of course, the painful left scars of shingles didn't help the itching on top of the sores that has spread all over my body. It has been seven long years of hell and I knew God was going to bring me out of the fire real soon and to bring deliverance of good health to me.

I would say:

God's Word is truth.
My health comes from the Lord.
Thank you Lord, for keeping me in my right mind
and your love in my heart.
I couldn't have made it without you!
I have been faithful.
Waiting on a miracle.
I will keep hope alive.
Waiting to receive the manifestation of healing right here on earth.
It's my season to be blessed.
I don't care what people think or say about my situation anymore...and,
Yes, maybe the outward appearance may not look so pretty,
but I'm still here smiling!

Chapter 9

THE OPERATION

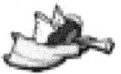

At 12:10 p.m. on July 18, 2007, I received a telephone call from Northwestern Memorial Hospital. At that time, my mother was at my home applying some ointment on my body to help relieve the itching. When the nurse confirmed that I was Dorothy Dearring she said, "We have a match for a liver transplant."

She said a child had received a portion of the same liver that morning through a split liver procedure with the same blood type and that there was enough for my transplant. She went on to say how my liver would regenerate and grow back to its normal size.

I thought I was dreaming; but believing in the impossible. My liver is here! At first, it was hard to believe. I paused and looked at my mother. I had took a deep breath; waiting to exhale my healing. My mother looked at me and I looked back at her. We couldn't believe it at first.

I called my fiancé to tell him the good news and he rushed over, rejoicing in the happy news. It was hard to swallow in my confused state-of-mind. I was so sleepy I wasn't thinking straight. The Holy Spirit spoke to me, "Wake up Dot, this is your season to be blessed. Shake it off! Your liver is here! Get excited about your miracle." I was overwhelmed with excitement.

I asked the nurse, "What should I do?"

"Look, wait by the phone and I'll call you right back to make sure it is a match within five minutes," she said.

I was filled with joy and laughter. In my heart, I knew it was a match.

She quickly called back and said, "Miss Dearring, it's a match. How soon can you get here?"

"Right now," I said. "I have to phone my dad to find out how soon we can get on the highway."

At that moment, my mother seemed to have a little fear and sadness on her face. "Mom, I got my liver! Thank you God, for my liver! I assured her, "You have nothing to worry about or be concern of, it is going to be alright in Jesus name. Just pray for me."

> *For the joy of the Lord is your strength.*
> Nehemiah 8:10

My joy gave me strength and I begin rejoicing the Lord with a shout of worship. My mother thought I was acting a little silly, but I was getting my praise on to get what God had for me—my liver! I am not holding anything back; I didn't care what she thought. Otherwise, she will never understand why I praise the Lord the way I do.

Until the day, she accepts the Lord as her personal savior in her *heart* and has a *relationship* with HIM, and then she would know why I praise God. She embraced me with a big hug, a tender kiss and told me how much she loved me.

She said, "I will pray that the surgery goes well, daughter."

"Look Mom, God got this!" She smiled as she headed towards the door to go home.

Soon after she left, Calvin and I prayed and rejoiced together in Jesus' Name. He gently kissed me with loving affection and gave me a big Holy hug. He let me know God loved me and God had my back!

"Yes, honey I got this," I replied. "I cannot wait when it is all said and done. I can't wait to feel good and live again."

After Calvin left, I had to get ready and prepare spiritually, physically and mentally for the trip to Northwestern Memorial Hospital. I call Ethel to let her know that the hospital had phoned me about the liver transplant match. She said Dad was playing golf and I had to call him on his cell phone to tell him the good news.

"Hello, Daddy, guess what? Daddy, I got my new liver!"

"What!" he said.

"Yes, Daddy, we need to get ready and go to Chicago as soon as possible to do a liver transplant."

"To God be the glory!" he said.

My dad was so overwhelmed and excited that he had one of his friend drive him back in a golf cart to get his car. I was very excited and a little nervous. I called my Bishop and his wife, then my supervisors Fred Elizondo and Jeff VandenBoss. (The one thing I was not going to allow was fear to come into my mind).

After that, I called Mrs. Doris Dearring, Georgia Howard, my best girls Michelle Franklin, Esther Hardin, Jeanette Payne, Jeanette Broadway (Nippy), Marilyn Morris, Mary Cusic, Linda Burnside, Meria Wyrick, and Victoria Tibbs. I asked everyone to keep us in prayer for a safe drive and surgery.

Mother Judith Jones quickly connected with other people who she knew through her email asking for urgent prayer for me. Coworkers at the Federal Centers were connecting with others in prayer for me too. I hurried and called my aunt Violet Kelly in Detroit to pray for me; my beautiful cousin, Dr. Janice Holmes, had her church to pray for me; my aunt Mary Smith in Thompson, GA, her lovely daughter, Edith Harvey, and other relatives in Georgia too, "keep us all up in prayer." And the prayer line went on and on, praying and believing that God will answer our prayers.

The Operation

As I rushed to get dressed, the nurse phoned back wondering if I had left my home yet. I told her I was waiting on my dad to pick me up and she stressed the urgency for me to get there quickly. I asked if I needed to bring anything with me, she laughed, "No, just your body!"

In the back of my mind, I needed to clean up my house and I thought of all kinds of excuses for not wanting to go to Chicago.

"Why now?" I said. Then, I took a step back and slowly exhaled. As I sat down to dress myself I thought, it's over! I guess I will not be skinny any longer—for the first time in my life, I enjoyed wearing petite clothing. They are so much cheaper to buy. Oh well, I did look rather cute in them and it was fun while it lasted. That's life! But this itching got to go in Jesus' name. I begin to speak authority over my body and to my spirit:

So then faith cometh by hearing, and hearing by the word of God.
Romans 10:17

For we walk by faith, not by sight.
II Corinthians 5:7

Heal me, O Lord, and I shall be healed; save me, and I shall be saved: for thou art my praise.
Jeremiah 17:14

For I will restore health unto thee, and I will heal thee of thy wounds, saith the Lord.
Jeremiah 30:17

Therefore I give no place to sickness or pain. So shall my word be that goeth forth out of my mouth: it shall not return unto me void, but it shall accomplish that which I please, and it shall prosper in the thing whereto I sent it. Isaiah 55:11

At that moment, I did not even have an appetite; I was too excited about getting my liver. Ethel called back and told me she was still waiting for my dad while she was packing and throwing her clothes, toothbrush, etc. in a travel bag. Once he got home and packed, he called me to see if I was ready.

"Not yet Dad?"

He called back about ten minutes later and asked again, "Are you ready yet Dot?"

"Almost, Daddy." I was getting a little frightened and I didn't know why. My mind was telling me, *No*, and my soul was saying, *You need to get your act together and go get your liver. What are you waiting on?* I prayed, for enough strength, and I was ready. I call my dad and he said, "Amen, she finally ready."

When I looked up to heaven as my dad was driving, I knew then that everything was turning around in my life. In all my struggles, challenges and issues I could start to live again, healthy! It is a shame that we weren't going shopping or to see Oprah and tell my healing story of inspiration. One day, she will hear about my story, because I will live to tell it! "There is no fear in love; but perfect love casteth out fear: because fear hath torment. He that feareth is not made perfect in love" (I John 4:18).

> *He sent his word, and healed them,*
> *and delivered them their destructions.*
> Psalm 107:20

In the back seat, I said a silent prayer to God. While my dad kept his eyes focused on the highway, Ethel was quietly sitting in the passenger seat. My heart was beating rapidly and I was praying at the same time. I was mediating on God's Word and thinking about when it is all over. In my heart, deep down in the depth of my soul, I knew I was going to be all right in Jesus' name, because I never lost my faith in God.

I began to speak scriptures:

> *I shall not die, but live, and declare the works of the Lord.*
> Psalm 118:17

> *Trust in the Lord with all thine heart;*
> *and lean not unto thine own understanding.*
> Proverbs 3:5

> *Let not your heart be troubled: ye believe in God,*
> *believe also in me.*
> John 14:1

> *I can do all things in Jesus Christ that strengthen me.*
> Philippians 4:13

> *And we know that all thing work together for good to them that love*
> *God, to them who are the called according to His purpose.*
> Romans 8:28

For some Godly reason, we were in Chicago in less than two hours (depending on the traffic it could take up to three hours). It did not seem real. It was as if we were floating on a heavenly cloud, sailing with God. It was almost as if God had divided and open up the highway like the Red Sea as he did for Moses and the people of Israel.

As I looked behind us, it seemed like we were the only cars on the highway. There was no backed-up construction traffic, no accidents, or flat tire to fix along the way. It was amazing! God had everything under control and knew how important it was for me to get to Chicago safely.

He knew how much time I had to get to the hospital, because the liver has a length of time to be kept frozen. The ride was the most joyous, marvelous, smooth sailing ride that I had been on in a long time. I would always remember that moment for the rest of my life.

Once we arrived at Northwestern Memorial Hospital, we had to enter on the second floor because after 5 p.m. the front entrance doors would be locked. After my dad swooped into the parking lot and parked, he rushed to find a rest room and Ethel was trying to keep up with him. As for me, I pressed on slowly not far behind them both. Within a blink of an eye, Dad went another direction to rush to the men's room. Ethel and I walked through the entrance doors as they opened up.

As he headed straight toward the rest room, we saw my dad coming up on the elevator.

He said, "How did you two get in here?" He was confused because the entrance door we came into was supposed to be locked. He said he had tried to get through the main doors but they were locked, making him go another direction up the elevator and back around to where we were.

Ethel and I laughed. "Well, what can we say Daddy? We had no problem walking through the second floor entrance doors as if someone had open up for us. I guess we got it like that!" I said.

Finally, we made it to the front desk. They called a nurse to come down to wheel me to the 17th floor. As we, all rode the elevator, a woman in the elevator had a take-out order of rib tips, collard greens, and the works. I wanted to ask her if I could try a taste. After smelling the food, I remembered I hadn't eaten anything at all. I asked the coordinator, if I could go straight back down to the second floor cafeteria to order me something to eat.

"You're kidding me," the coordinator laughed, and my dad and Ethel joined in. The coordinator said, "It is a good thing that you haven't eaten because you are getting ready to go into surgery."

Everything moved quickly. The transplant team confirmed the liver was a match. I could hear God say, "This is your season, your miracle, my blessing, and a second chance with a new gift of life!"

Wow! I felt good. I had kept the faith and put only my trust in God. Not only was the liver for me, but a child had received a portion as well—a double blessing of life.

The coordinator nurse asked me many questions while they were preparing me for surgery. I had to change into a hospital gown and step on the scale to get my weight. My dad and Ethel were praying before it was time for my surgery. Within ten minutes, a young man came to take my dad and Ethel to the seventh floor to wait.

The Kovler Organ Transplant program of Northwestern Memorial Hospital had made arrangements. The suites are provided for transplant patients and their caregivers who live a far distance from Northwestern Memorial Hospital. It provides them with convenient access to any necessary outpatient care needed for approximately two to three weeks. Later that evening, the hospital assigned daddy and Ethel to a hotel in a temporary housing program for recovery patients at Marriott Residence Hotel.

Then finally, another nurse walked into the room with a bed I was to transfer onto. There was no time to talk, to breathe or to do anything. Ready or not the transplant team had their work cut out in Jesus' Name. Yes, I am getting my liver!

Soon the nurse gave me papers to sign permission to do the surgery. My whole heart seemed to drop quickly down to my stomach. I had taken some deep breaths, inhaled and exhaled quietly. This is what I have been waiting on for seven years.

"Did I need to see a priest before I go into surgery?" she asked.

"No, I have the Most High God right here by my side, but thanks anywhere," I said kindly.

She smiled and left the room. My dad, Ethel, and I held hands to pray for the preparation before it was time for my surgery. In about five minutes, two nurses came to the room to help prep me with an IV, and a pill to calm my nervous stomach. Before I knew it, my eyes were getting heavy, I started to get very sleepy. The other nurse grabbed the bed and wheeled me to the transplant surgical floor where the operation will be taken place. I told my parents I loved them both. They both said how much they appreciate and love me too.

I couldn't turn back or look back on my circumstances, situations, or condition at that moment. The only thing that was on my mind was *Oh Almightily, Heavenly Father, Oh Jehovah, and my Creator.* I could have gone on and on praising the Lord at that moment. I *love* the word of God and life that gives me life more abundantly.

When I gave my *heart* to God, all the glory and victory goes to Him. If it was not for the Lord on my side, I could not have made it. Sometime I do not understand how or why some people choose to live day after day and not know the Almighty King! Thank God, I'm covered in the blood, in Jesus' Name. The most precious gift I could ever have in this life is the Holy Spirit–it's priceless. The thrill of it all! With *all my heart*, I will glorify your name *forever*. I know Almighty God, got a *blessing* with my name on it, and I came to Chicago, Illinois to get it!

So then faith cometh by hearing, and hearing by the Word of God.
Romans 10:17

A liver transplant is an operation that replaces a patient's diseased liver with a whole or partial healthy liver from another person. Liver transplantation surgery is a complicated process. There are really three operations. The first is the removal of the liver from the donor. If the liver is donated at a different location, it must be transferred to the transplant center under sterile refrigerated conditions within 24 hours. The second operation is the removal of the diseased liver from the patient, and the third is the operation to insert and connect to the new liver. The operations on the recipients are so detailed they require a long time to complete. The team of surgeons, nurses, and support staff, are now very experienced in the technique.

The Operation

The right lobe of the liver is about 60% of the liver, leaving 40% of a normal liver in the donor. Because of its amazing capacity to regenerate, the liver is restored to its original size in the donor and grows to a comparable size in the recipient, in approximately four weeks.

Anytime there is a donor operation that comes from an individual, it typically takes between four and eight hours, but may vary depending on your anatomy and any previous abdominal surgeries you may have had. From the recovery room, you will then be taken to a hospital bed on the fifth floor. Any family members or friends were allowed to visit during regular hospital visitation hours, which were from 8 a.m. to 8 p.m.

Once the surgery is completed, I was taken immediately from the operating room to the recovery room where I waken from the anesthesia. I opened my eyes on July 18, 2007, after a five and half hour operation. Thank God, I am healthy again! As I was recuperating, my spiritual ears heard my dad and Ethel's voices as they were waiting for me to wake up. "That the trial of your faith, being much more precious than of gold that perisheth, though it be tried with fire, might be found unto praise and honour and glory at the appearing of Jesus Christ" (I Corinthians 14:33).

After the surgery, all I could do was smile. I still felt a little woozy from the medication, but was glad to be alive. I tried to move around, but the nurses had to calm me down, to stay still. *Thank you Jesus, I make it!* I could not help it but to get excited! I tried to talk and shout for joy, "Praises God, I got my miracle!"

A tube was inserted through my nose down into my throat and into my stomach. The tube was only temporary but helped keep the stomach empty to help prevent nausea and vomiting. A Foley catheter had been inserted to monitor my urine output closely. This catheter felt slightly uncomfortable, but it was only temporary and would be remove when I was able to get out of bed safely to urinate on my own. While lying there, I waited as the nurses prepared to take me to another recovering room. I lay still and heard my dad joyful tears knowing that his baby girl make it through. Ethel quietly and peacefully rejoicing. I could feel the victory celebration in my spirit.

Their is one word most misunderstood and dreaded by new transplant recipients–rejection! Two of the most common complications following liver transplant are rejection and infection. Rejection most likely occurs during a period immediately after transplant, but may occur many years later for many reasons.

Still, I was slowly trying to speak. All I could do was to send a happy smile to heaven where I could hear God say, "Well done miracle daughter, you kept the faith." At that time, being still seemed impossible. I was so full of joy. Hallelujah!

It is a good feeling to stand on God's Word and faith. The physicians had taken out the old liver and God's miracle replaced a new liver so that I can live a healthy and normal life. Miracles do happen! There is nothing too little or too big for our heavenly Father. Now, you know, there is something behind that smile and a reason why I smile.

It is not a religious thing. It's a heart thing! It is having a relationship with God, learning to know Him for yourself; it is necessary to have Christian doctrine, teaching, facts, principles or beliefs, the gospel truth, the word of God, and the New Testament so that you learn your purpose's here on earth. It's a *heart* thing! How could anyone live without knowing the Lord? It is unbelievable!

> *For therein is the righteousness of God revealed from faith to faith; as it is written, the just shall live by faith.*
> Romans 1:17

Usually, the transplant team resolves complications through medication and/or surgery. The most common complications shortly after surgery are poor function of the new liver (primary graft failure), bleeding inside the body, bacterial infection and rejection of the liver.

The Operation

Later that day, I was taken back to the intensive care room for one or two days depending upon how sick, I was after the transplant surgery. Some reason, I was bleeding inside my body and losing a lot of blood. The nurse and physician had to find somewhere to stop the bleeding. They checked the level count and said it needs to be a little higher.

Note: Bleeding is a risk of any surgical procedure but a particular risk after liver transplantation because of the extensive nature of the surgery and because clotting requires factors made by the liver. Most transplant patients bleed a minor amount and may get additional transfusions after the operation. If bleeding is substantial or brisk, return to the operating room for control of the bleeding is often necessary. In general, approximately 10% of transplant recipients will require a second operation for bleeding.

I had one of the nurses call my parents back into my room. I explained what the doctors were thinking about doing; to take me back into surgery if the bleeding didn't stop. My dad and Ethel called on Jehovah, our Healer, our God that sees everything and provides are needs. We continued to pray and pray in Jesus Name. Finally, they both kissed me goodnight and said, "Trust in God, it's going to be alright, God hasn't failed you yet, daughter. He didn't bring you this far for nothing."

Throughout the night, until the early morning it was critical. I did not know if I had to go back into surgery because of the blood count that was very low. I prayed all day and night for the blood count levels to go above 7.0; it was necessary. The nurses were very helpful and kind. I was so helpless at that moment. All I could do was pray and called on Jesus. I was ready to go home to be with my family.

The nurse and physicians had to keep a close eye on my blood count, poking needles, continually drawing blood from my arm and taking medication to help prevent me from any infection. I recalled around 4:30 a.m., the nurses checked my blood work again. All night long, they were poking, bruising and drawing blood from my arm for a chance to see if the blood count had changed.

The nurse rushed back into my room with a happy smile. My blood count was 9.3. It started as low as 1.78 and it had gone above 7.0. Thank you, Jesus! Here I was rejoicing, joyfully and repeatedly with every raindrop of tears that came my way. Now, maybe I can get some rest! God blessed my miracle! And it did come too passed in Jesus' Name. (Later, I learned my liver came from a young person who died in an accident.)

Between 5:30-6:30 a.m., a young male nurse approached my bed and was ready to wheel me back into surgery. I quickly paused and quickly pushed myself to sit-up in the bed.

"We must take you right back into surgery now!" he ordered.

"Oh no, no…. I'm not going back in the operation room," I said.

"Miss Dearring, I'm only following doctor's orders."

"Look here, I have my own doctor's orders too," I said firmly. "My orders come from the most high, God! I'm healed and that is that!"

He was not too happy about that. This may had been too deep for him to swallow. I told him that the nurse replied to me earlier, no surgery. She said I was doing great; my blood count is 9.3. I will let the doctors know that as he checked the chart with her notes on it.

"I am very sorry, but you're doing great, no surgery!" he said apologizing. "What an awesome report."

"Yes, God is good! I added. "God has the last say. God is my healer, my provider and deliverance me from sickness!" We both smiled.

My girlfriend, Jeanette Payne quickly rode the train to Chicago to see how I was doing. At first, I could not believe it! Jeanette kept her word. She stayed there in the room with me until the next morning. I called it, "Love." Jeanette later went to the gift shop and bought me a

The Operation

beautiful musical stuffed brown bear clothed in a green shirt and hat with white pearls. This bear sung a song called, "That's What Friends Are For."

The next morning, the physician who did my surgery had a transplant team with him. They took a looked at my scar. It was beautiful!

One of the nurses said, "Oh doctor, Miss Dorothy will need to learn how to walk all over again. Yes, of course."

Then I realized that I had not packed any clothes from home. The only clothes I had was the ones I wore to Chicago hospital. As my health was rapidly increasing back normal, I had to get up out of bed to learn how to walk with a walker throughout the hallway of the hospital. My dad, Ethel, and Jeanette helped collect money so I could have medications to take after the surgery.

My dad went to the Walgreen's pharmacy inside the hospital to pick up the medications that came with a large tote bag. It contained all types of medications for liver transplant patients such as: Prednisone 5M tablets, Cellcept 250MG capsules, Prograf 1 MG twice daily, Pepcid 20MG, Bactrim SS Tablets, Nystatin 5cc = 1 TSP, Valcyte 450MG, Magnesium 450MG, Zoloft 200MG, Toprol 50MG, a thermometer and Upper Arm Blood Pressure Monitor and others.

Now that Jeanette knew that I was all right, she caught the train back home the next day. I did not want her to go!

I had to watch my blood pressure to make sure it would not go over 140,' and that my temperature didn't go over 101.5'. If that happened, I had to call the hospital as soon possible. As Ethel and a nurse went over all my medications slowly, they explained how to use them and really understand the names to each pill. The pharmacy included a pillbox organizer for each day of the week according to directions on the bottle.

I have never had to take so much medicine in my life. I thanked God for Ethel, because she was more familiar with medications then I was. She was very helpful. Recovering from a major surgery is the first step to feeling healthy, healing, and having a positive outlook–mentally and physically–to resume the normal activities in life.

I was taken to the transplant room on the fifth floor for approximately five days. During my recovery, I felt somewhat bloated. They had given me steroids that made my whole body blow up like a large beach ball. My weight tipped the scale at 164 pounds and I was trying to get back into size six skirt. I could not even get my right thigh in a small.

"Oh, my God, what happened?" I said loudly to myself.

Ethel actually heard me mumbling from the bathroom door. She heard me talking at the mirror as if I saw myself change into a spiritual bionic woman. As if, I was getting ready to fight the spiritual battles of earth. I called for love, joy, peace, kindness, hope and forgiveness in Jesus' name to stomp out the evil force of hate, envy, jealous, selfness, adultery, and lying.

Ethel heard me outside the door and she was chucking with tears heavy rolling down her cheeks. I was laughing too. Here I am strong and ready to fight Satan and take back what the enemy had stolen from me. I was going to get everything that belonged to me—my health, my finances, and living the good life that God promised me to have.

"There's no stopping me now!"

The Kovler Organ Transplant program of Northwestern Memorial Hospital had arranged for Dad and Ethel to stay at Marriott Residence hotel. Before I was discharged, I had been assigned to a temporary housing program for recovery patients before sending me back home. The suites are provided for transplant patients and their caregivers who live a far distance from Northwestern Memorial Hospital. It provides them with convenient access to any necessary outpatient care needed for approximately two to three weeks.

During the time, we stayed at the hotel to recovery my dad had driven back to Battle Creek to take care of some unfinished business. At the same time, I didn't have any clothes to wear, only the hospital gowns. I called mother Georgia Howard and Jeanette Payne to see if they could gather up some clothes for me to wear. They arrange a place and time to meet my dad to drop off the clothes that I needed. The clothes fit perfectly!

"That's what I called teamwork angels! Thank you so much from the bottom of my heart, mother Howard and Jeanette for all your help, I love you both dearly in Jesus Name."

It was a wonder that I was able to digest any of the different types of medicine that had to be taken with food or milk, and which ones not to take on an empty stomach. Thank God for Ethel! She was very loving and caring. One night, I had gotten so ill that Ethel began to pray. For a moment, Ethel thought she had to call the hospital, but I started to feel better. God says it is not over, until *He* says it is over!

My fiancé called my dad every day to see how I was doing after the surgery. After the recovery, I was able to talk to him. That following week, Calvin called and asked me, if I was still going to marry him now that I had my new liver? He wanted to set the date. I had promised him once I received my liver we would set a date. I could not go back on my word.

"What about doing it on July 18, 2009?" I asked.

"Yeah, sounds good!" he said.

The best thing in life comes at the most unexpected moments when you least expect it. It is good to *wait* on the Lord, for your unexpected moments. Throughout the weeks at the hotel, they provided free breakfast, lunch and dinner expect on the weekends. Some weekends my mother would cook Ethel and me a delicious meal for my dad to bring back to Chicago. Ethel took excellent care of me and we enjoyed each other's company.

My girlfriend, Jewel Thomas called to see how I was doing. She asked, "If there is anything I needed?" At first, I hesitated and did not know how to respond. Therefore, I swallow my pride because my money was getting low. Jewell collected a donation from the coworkers and friends to help me with the medications, food etc., that I needed.

"Oh boy, that took a weight off my shoulder," I said.

"All, you have to do is ask, we love you Dot," she said.

It looked as everything was beginning to fall back in place with my health, as if I had not been though a storm of life. My hair was growing back. sores were disappearing.

"Oh yes, no more itching! Hallelujah! Hallelujah! Praise the Lord!"

God is good! He sees everything and knows your heart. It is how you live your life that shines. Treat others as you want to be treated, with *respect and love.*

> *And ye shall seek me, and find me, when ye shall search for me with all your heart.*
> Jeremiah 29:13

Chapter 10

THERE'S NO PLACE LIKE HOME

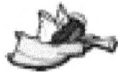

August 08, 2007

When the hospital released me to go home, my neighbors greeted me with a smile and a friendly wave. Val Mabry was very glad to see me back home in Jesus' name. At first, I was nervous at the thought of getting out of my dad's van. I could not wait to get back home to be around family and friends. Ethel and I had been together almost two months in Chicago. She truly had taken good care of me as if she had given birth to me. I believe not too many stepmothers would have done what she did in Jesus' Name.

Home sweet home, there's no place like home.

I used my walker to enter my home. There was my mother, daughter Nicole, and grandchildren Jasmine, Juan, and Joshua waiting inside with a warm welcome home. My grandchildren had made me a lovely poster and let me know how much they had missed their grandmother. The first thing that came out there mouth was, "Are you still itching?"

"Heavens, No!" I said.

They all shouted for joy and gave me hugs and kisses. One of my neighbors stopped by the house and expressed that I shouldn't be doing too much of anything, but to get plenty rest to heal. She offered to be of assistance if I needed it.

My testimony one day will be the greatest story ever written from generation to generation to come. I pray that my testimony will bless someone that is going through a difficult time and can be inspired by a story written about a liver transplant. I'm a walking, living, *testimony*, because I am alive. Today and every day, when I wake up and think about the goodness of the Lord I get so excited knowing that I am still here! I am so glad that I didn't1 wait until something truly could have happened to me before I sought the Lord. You see, I'm saved by the blood, anointed, and have a covenant relationship with God.

For the rest of my life, I will praise the Lord and serve Him. There's no looking back, keep it moving forward in Him. The Lord has a purpose for my life. That is why I am alive!

Satan tried to attack my faith, steal my joy, and destroy my physical body. He wanted me died when I accepted the Lord as my personal Savior and gave my *heart* and life to God. I never looked back because there was nothing to look back on but drama and trouble. Satan will come to attack Christians even harder. Unbelievably, Satan is working overtime to get us to go back into the world in sin. That is Satan's job description making constant accusations against the people of God.

> *For God is not the author of confusion, but of peace.*
> I Corinthians 14:33

I selected the wrong men in my life thinking that they were the best thing that could have happend to me. But God was not in it at all. God was always in my heart and He healed my broken heart when I made the wrong choice of men.

Each day I grabbed *faith*, grabbed *trusting* God, grabbed *believing*, and grabbed *keeping* hope alive in my *heart*. Everyone will go through *the trials of life*-you cannot doubt faith—whether it is sickness or a broken heart. Who will you grab when sickness attacks your body, your finances, broken relationships, or unhappy heart?

I will hold on to God's word because I have a divine appointment and destiny for a blessing in Him.

> *You therefore, my son, be strong in the grace that is in Christ Jesus.*
> II Timothy 2:1

If you didn't know, now you know. There is a man who I chose to be with for the rest of my life. He is my *first* love. He understands our pain and he is one of a kind. He sees me as *royalty* and a *queen*. I get so excited when I hear his name. I put my trust in him, my faith, my joy, and my whole heart belongs to him.

He never holds a grudge in his heart; if you make a mistake, he knows how to forgive. He will not break your heart or spirit. He cares and shows kindness, because he is love. He does not believe in emotional or verbal abuse, and you will never have to think if he is talking about you behind your back.

His love is unconditional and real. He adores you; he will *never* leave you nor forsake you. He knows your strength and weakness. He is a man of peace and good. The man who I am describing is compassionate and loves me. His name is Jesus. I dare you to try him!

> *And we have known and believed the love that God hath to us. God is love; and he that dwelleth in love dewlleth in God, and God in him.*
> I John 4:16

On August 11, 2008, my lovely future sister-in-law, Meria Wyrick drove me to Chicago for a follow-up at the hospital. My financé Calvin, rode with us. I enjoyed going to Chicago, but wished it were under difference circumstance. Instead, of going to the hospital, I wished we were going shopping at Macy's, visiting the Johnson's magazine offices, or seeing *The Oprah Winfrey Show* as an author. Oprah is someone I have always loved to meet. I can only dream and hope to see her in person one day, and introduce my first book to her book club.

Once we arrived at Northwestern Memorial Hospital, I couldn't wait for everyone to see the new me. As we approach the elevator doors to go to the 17th floor. I signed in and one of the nurses was pleased to see how fabulous I looked. Some of them were filled with tears of joy, laughing, hugging, and saying, "Look at God!" One of the staff members was shocked to hear that it had only been a year since my transplant. She thought I had my surgery done about three or five years ago because of how well I had adjusted.

My doctor, J. Leskiseky was very pleased to see how well I was doing. His response was, "Wow!" You know this was phenomenal!"

Yes, doctors call it phenomenal. I called it, believed and received my healing in faith. "I shall not die, but live, and declare the works of the Lord" (Psalms 118:17).

The definition of *Phenomenal:* Very good or great; Something absolutely fantastic and one of a kind in greatness; Extraordinary, highly unusual or relating to the unexplained or supernatural. From a Greek root meaning, "appearance," phenomenal describes something so awesome and borderline miraculous.

No one in the world should ever experience this kind of sickness. The itching alone was enough to make you want to lose your mind. I never gave up wanting to live the good life that God promised me. Through it all, I let go and gave it to God. He said, "Dorothy, Well done!" I was created for God's glory, to love Him, to worship Him, to serve Him, and to know Him for myself. I got the *victory* in Jesus' name!

> *Now faith is the substance of things hoped for,*
> *the evidence of things not seen.*
> Hebrews 11:1

Today I'm only taking one medication, Prograf. I know that one day, down the road, I may not be taking them either. I can be medication free, in Jesus' name! I asked myself how I felt about having a transplant before the surgery and after? Now that I'm healed, how did it benefit my life? Well, the answer to that is, it is almost as if I had to plead to the board of hospital to make a decision to understand how *serious* my condition was. It was *prayer, faith, favor* and God that helped move me from the bottom of the list to the top while my doctor was submitting letters to board of directors.

The Spirit Filled Life Bible for Students stated, (Genesis 22:12-14), the test of *Faith* shows, God always *tests faith* to see if it is pure and strong. Trials and tribulations are part of life; everyone has them. I would not have made it, if I did not have stand patiently and believe in God's word.

> *God is not a man that he should lie; neither the son of man that he should repent: hath he said, and shall he not do it? Or hath he spoken, and shall he not make it good? Behold, I have received commandment to bless: and he hath blessed; and I cannot reverse it.*
> Numbers 23:19-20

I knew God was going to heal me if I spoke healing and scriptures out my mouth, mixed it with faith, and believed. If I had spoken sickness all the time, that's what I would have had. I spoke healing, and I could have whatever I said. During the seven years of my illness, I spoke *healing* every day, even though my body was ill.

On July 18, 2014, I *celebrated* the seven-year anniversary of my liver transplant. Now you know the reason why I have something to smile about…and I'm looking forward many more years smiling in Jesus' name.

> *And we know that all things work together for good to them that love God, to them who called according to His purpose.*
> Romans 8:28

Where is your faith? Jesus was trying to teach His followers to trust Him completely, even when things got rough, Jesus is in control. He "rebuked the wind and the raging of the water" with spiritual authority. Jesus did not give in to the circumstances. Instead, He took authority over them! You must have *faith* in our Christian walk. You cannot have any doubt, when you are living for the Lord. You have to believe in Him.

For we walk by faith, not by sight.
II Corinthians 5:7

A transplant is more than an operation; it is an experience that will affect you the rest of your life. At first, you will make changes so your body can recuperate from the surgery and effects of liver disease. As you recover further, you can resume most normal activities. However, some lifestyle changes may be long term. For example, you must adjust to a strict medication routine and must be more cautious about matters like catching a cold.

Treatment does not end when you leave the medical center. Outpatient follow-up is an important part of your care...for the rest of your life. Once you leave the hospital, you will still need many medical check-ups. Every three months, I would go to the Regional Lab in Battle Creek for blood work. They would forward the result back to Northwestern Memorial Hospital.

Liver transplantation is an important move forward in the treatment of severe liver disease. It has opened a new world for patients who otherwise were destined to die from their liver disease. The operation is a major one, and there are still problems associated with medications used to prevent rejection. But overall, patients can usually expect a good outcome with return to normal activities.

And he that searcheth the hearts knoweth what is the mid of the Spirit, because he maketh intercession for the saints according to the will of God.
And we know that all things work together for good to them that love God, to them who are the called according to his purpose.
Romans 8:27-28

But seek ye first the kingdom of God and his righteousness and all these things shall be added unto you.

Matthew 6:33

Chapter 11

THE WEDDING: TWO HEARTS, ONE LOVE

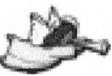

On July 17, 2009, everyone in the wedding party had to meet at the church by 6 p.m. for the rehearsal dinner. It was a lovely and hot evening. Kathy's Catering brought food for the wedding party. The photographer, Edward Hooks, Sr. and his lovely wife, Dee Hooks had also attended. Connie Williams was there to help on the audio system for the songs that needs to be played for the wedding—especially, "Here Comes the Bride."

Aunt Juliette Tyler (on Calvin's side of the family) and his lovely niece Charmia Wyrick, also helped decorate the church. Everyone involved in the wedding party played a part. My two best girls, Michelle Franklin and Esther Harden, helped prepared the table, and Esther's neighbor, Laura prepared a fruit salad that was appetizing and scrumptious.

After the rehearsal dinner, some sad news spread quickly throughout the church. The best man, Leodis Williams (Calvin's cousin) had learned that his stepson had been shot. He left and our hearts went out to him. At this point, it was very difficultly to continue the wedding party; all we could do was pray and hope that he was still alive.

July 18, 2009, was our wedding day. At around 6:15 a.m., I had got on my knees and said my morning prayers, "Lord, you are still in control, today is the day, everything will be all right, in Jesus' name. Lord, I asked that you give the wedding party favor, strength, and joy on this day in Jesus' name. Touch each and every one's heart as we begin this journey as Mr. and Mrs. Calvin L. Wyrick." What a lovely sound!

I never thought I would be getting married once again. My dream to be a bride had come true. I called it, "My Spiritual Wedding of the 21th Century!" This was my second marriage and I knew this time

God was in it; it was in season and had His blessing. God pleasantly placed Calvin in my life when I was so seriously ill. Calvin kept coming back, knocking on my door. At the time of my trials, I felted I was not attractive enough to have a man.

Calvin had told me long before the wedding that, all he wanted was my heart. He knew once God healed, God was going to restored me back to what I used to look like as if nothing had happen. Calvin knew of my condition before the transplant, and that I didn't have time for any man, period! All I was doing was waiting on my miracle. And now, today, this moment of my life, I was getting ready to share a part of my life with a *handsome king*.

On our wedding day, it turned out to be a little cool and dreary. But it wouldn't even matter. I was still going to marry my man! I could not wait for the wedding party to come stepping out into the sanctuary with our favorite song, "Only You Can Make Me Happy," by Surface. Our song, "Heaven Sent," by Alise Cole, was also on the list.

I packed and loaded all the decorations into my car to take to Comfort Inn hotel for the reception. As I rushed around, news spread through the city that the stepson (who had been shot the night before) had passed away. I didn't know what to do. Should Calvin and I go ahead with the wedding or cancel it?

This was tragic and painful news to hear about a young man who had an electrifying smile and a warm heart. He always had a kind word to cheer both family, friends, and was an outstanding athlete and performer at Battle Creek Central High School. Why did this happen? This day would always be a reminder of this horrible news and the loss of Dominique.

Once I arrived at the Comfort Inn, my two dearest cousins, Kristena and Charlene Drain, came to help set up for the reception. When I entered the banquet room, I was devastated that the place was not cleaned from the night before. There I stood, quietly frustrated, hurt, and teary eyed. I had to try to get my thoughts together, and to unload the boxes of decorations.

Deep inside my soul was crushed and unhappy with the condition of the room. I knew I had to be strong and not be a quitter, and to continue what I had set out to do...to have a wonderful and blessed day. I sat down for a few minutes to gather my thoughts. I was not going to let the devil steal my joy! Life is good, and too short to worry about the little things that were trying to bring my spirit down. Kristena reached out to grip my hand so we could take the time to pray. It worked!

We got started and I continued with my plans. I had a noon hair appointment and we still needed to set up tables and put up the decorations. Calvin's sister, Teresa and fiancé, Bo Brooks, arrived to help vacuum and set up the audio system. My grandchildren Juan and Joshua came to help take down chairs and put decorations on the tables. Everything was coming together nicely and I left for my hair appointment knowing things was in good hands.

Although I arrived thirty minutes early to my appointment, Nate, my hairdresser, was finishing up with my two best girls, Michelle and Esther. At that moment, all I could think was, I was going to be late to my own wedding. I left the hairdressers about 2 p.m. and headed straight home. I quickly jumped in the shower. In a couple hours I would be married.

Who so find a wife find a good thing,
obtained favor of the Lord.
Proverb 18:22

At about 2:15 p.m., Cathy, who altered my wedding dress, called and asked if I needed help getting into my dress? "Yes, please!" I said.

Thanks to all who made our wedding day a day to remember! Calvin and I express our heartfelt thanks to you, our families and friends, for celebrating with us the freshness of a new life, new beginnings, and new love as we exchange wedding vows. It's a Marriage– Heaven Sent.

The Wedding: Two Hearts, On Love

Bride: Dorothy M. Dearring
Groom: Calvin L. Wyrick
Minister: Bishop Hugh D. Smith, Jr
Maids-of-Honor: Ola Hughes (Bride's sister), and Meria Wyrick (Calvin's twin sister)
Bride's Maids: Nicole Mann (Bride's daughter), Channel Wyrick (Calvin's daughter), Esther Harden (Bride's best girl), Michelle Franklin (Bride's best girl), Kathy Mabry (Bride's cousin), and Charmia Wyrick (Calvin's niece)
Flower Girl: RaMyiah Renae Cooper (Bride's sister Ola's niece)
Best Man: Leodis Williams (Calvin's cousin)
Groom's Men: Terry Trust (Calvin's cousin), Charles C. Colen Jr., (Calvin's nephew), Christopher King (Bride's nephew), Marquis Jackson (Calvin's son), Lonnie Edwards (my cousin), and Michael Hightower (Calvin's cousin)
Ring Bearers: Juan Warren II and Joshua Mann (Bride's grandsons)
Hostesses: Tracey Hodges and Shawna Earl (Bride's stepsisters)
Soloist: Pastor J.C. Oliver
Photographer: Edward T. Hooks, Sr - Poppi Rome Picture Studio
Caterer: Kathy's Catering
Wedding Cake Design: Rose Richardson
Hair Stylist: Nate Johnson
Wedding Directors: Kim Parker and Angela J. Johnson-Patton

So these three things will last forever-
faith, hope, and love—and the greatest of these is love.
I Corinthians 13:13

That day was not only a celebration of two hearts coming together as one, it was a gift of hope, a second chance of life, a miracle from God. Two years after the liver transplant, the queen was marrying her king!

On our wedding day, God's love was going to show up in the sight of our families and friends, in the presence of His blessing. The clock struck 3 p.m., but the wedding didn't begin until 3:30 p.m. As the music and wedding party began, Bishop and Calvin waited on me. I begin to feel nervous and trembled all over.

I was excited to get down the aisle with my dad, and be married to my king. Once I approach the church sanctuary door entrance to walk down the aisle, I locked arms with my dad. I felt some nervousness but tried not to show it.

As I focused straight ahead, I saw what a chocolate, sexy man I was going to marry. He stood next to his best man, and the Bishop was smiling along with everyone in the wedding party. It was such a lovely sight to see. I will never forget that Kodak moment for the rest of my life! As I looked around the church, it was packed full of smiles with wonderful families and friends.

As Calvin and I lit the Unity candle together, we joined as one in Jesus' Name. What a powerful, anointed voice from a man of God, Pastor J. C. Oliver who sang, "When a Man Loves a Woman." It brought my teary eyes to a smile. "Loved it!"

After the wedding, my sister Ola, told my girlfriends, "I thank God…. that I didn't have to go to a funeral, but I am blessed to be going to my sister's wedding." Amen

That he would grant you, according to the riches of his glory, to be-
strengthened with might by his Spirit in the inner man;
That Christ may dwell in your hearts by faith; that ye,
being rooted and grounded in love.
Ephesians 3:16-17

In conclusion, writing this book has allowed me to tell the world about a unique and heartfelt style of my life. I had to bless the world by expressing the love of Christ. Not everyone is a liar or fake! The truth is, some people cannot accept someone who is *real*. How you live your life, and the choices you make, may come back to bite later down the road, if you are not careful.

Just do right and God will give it back to you by the way you touch other people's lives. I was so surprise by all the people I had touched through my *spirit of love*—you cannot even image. Yes, the haters do not like it. That is not going to keep me from being who God created me to be. And let it be written, "God is the only one that has kept me *happy* all my life; not a man.

It is a relationship to know Him for yourself. Only God knows our heart and only God can put happiness in it; men nor women can make us happy. I was created in His image to send you a smile and love your way, because there *is* something behind that smile. Now you know, I was born to be happy in Jesus Name!"

If you don't have a church home, I would love to invite you to come and attend our service at Emmanuel Covenant Church International, 585 Hubbard St, Battle Creek, MI, 49037, Dr. Senior Pastor Frederick J. Sweet and Co-Pastor Shannon Sweet at 11 a.m., Sunday morning, Sunday school at 9:30 a.m. We welcome you warmly in Jesus love.

Towards the end, when it all said and done, everyone's hearts will only be recognized in God's sight eternity. It's a heart thing!" For the moment, can we forgive? Can you forget? Can you say it is going to be all right? Can you take a friend in your arms and embrace them? Can you give yourself a hug or a pat on the back and find out that you are beautiful, special, precious, marvelous, fantastic and loving?

Knowing in this entire world, no one person is the same who God created; each one of us is unique! Whatever happens to people's sense of humor? It seems some people are more uptight about any little thing;

stressing over financial, their jobs, and children. "Get a grip, get Jesus!" Life is not that serious. Be thankful, you wake-up in your right mind; you have your health and strength and you still here! It seems some of us have forgotten how to laugh, smile and enjoy today's moments.

I never recognized who I was at a young age. I only wanted to fit in and be accepted by others to be liked. When God showed up in my life, his intention for me was to be a blessing to others by sending a smile. God accepts us for who we are, regardless of what people think. You are blessed in your own special way; just be real! Everyone should count their daily blessing, whether you connected or not with HIM. God loves you.

Beloved, let us love one another: for love is of God;
and every one loveth is born of God, and knowth God.
He that loveth not knoweth not God; for God is love.
I John 4:7-8

It's because of you Lord, that I was brought out of sickness. I wanted HIM to said, "Well, done my faithful servant!" Now, that my mind is made up, I will never go back! Through it all, I had grace to go through it, with a smile!

When we dedicate our life to Christ, we become a servant, to serve Him by helping others and to find our purpose. That is why I'm still here; to fulfill God's assignment here on earth, in Jesus' Name.

Use your gifts from God mindfully. Too many people leave this world taking their talents–unnoticed–with them to the grave. Prayer changes lives. I pray that my book has blessed you, inspires you about my healing and a man named Jesus...He's 100% Real! In 2016, I am a walking miracle. Look what God has done for me. He can do it for you, if you believe!

It is even a vapor that appeared for a
little time and then vanished away.
James 4:14

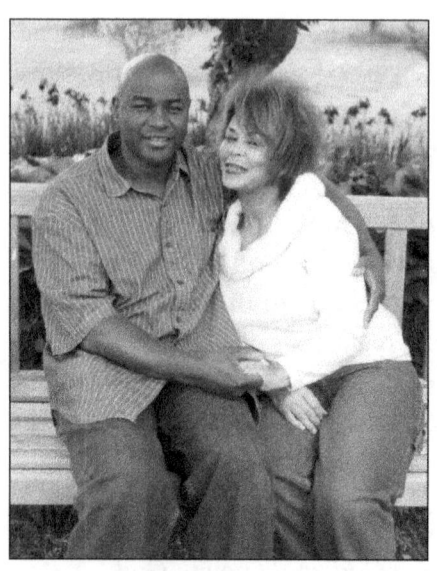
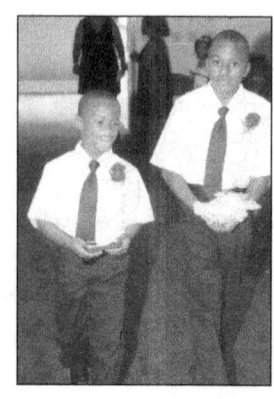
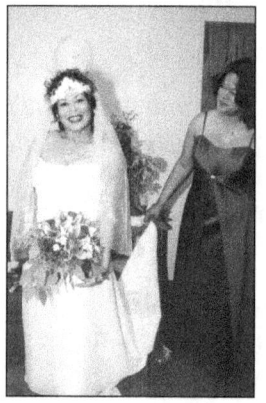
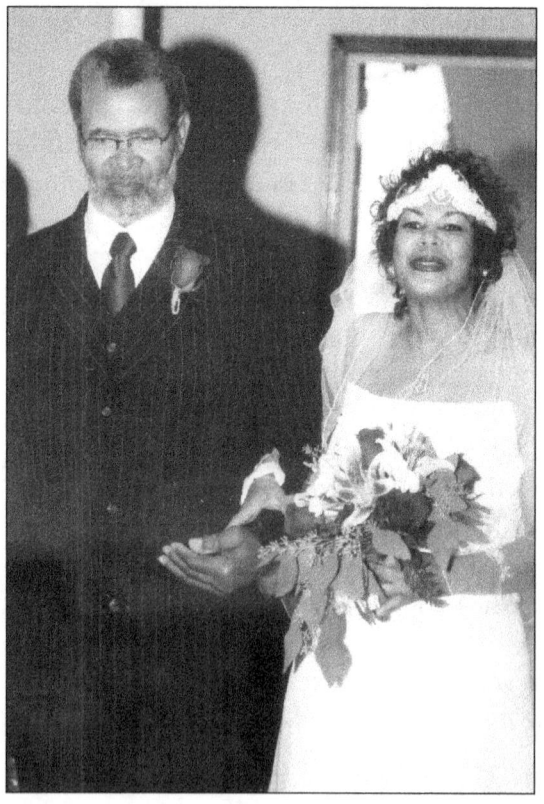

Clockwise: My grandsons, Juan Warren II and Joshua Mann were my ring bearers; my friend, Meria Wyrick-Colen helps me get ready for the big day; My father, Willie Mann Jr. was by my side throughout my entire illness, and now was able to walk his daughter down the isle; Calvin Wyrick and me during our engagement after my transplant.

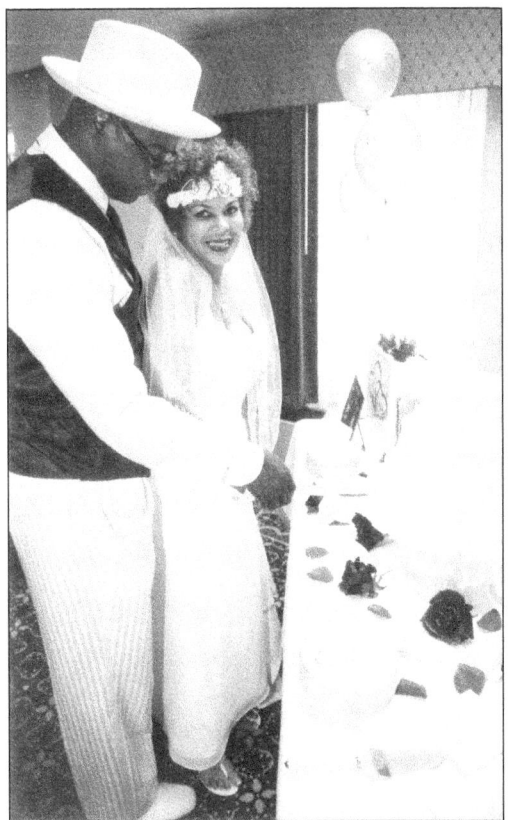
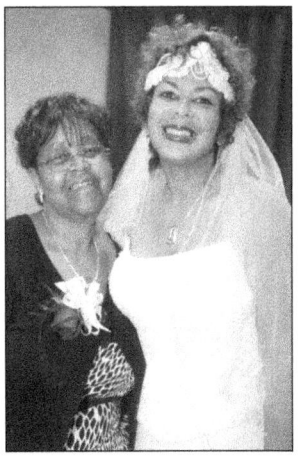
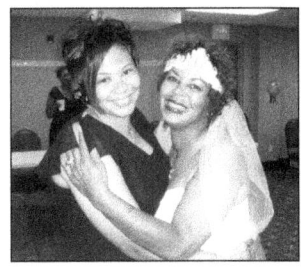
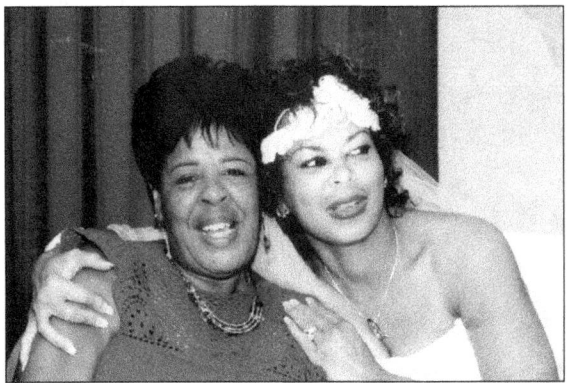

Clockwise: ; My mother Ola Mann and me; my daughter Nicole and me; my friend Jeanette Payne and me; and Calvin and I cut our wedding cake.

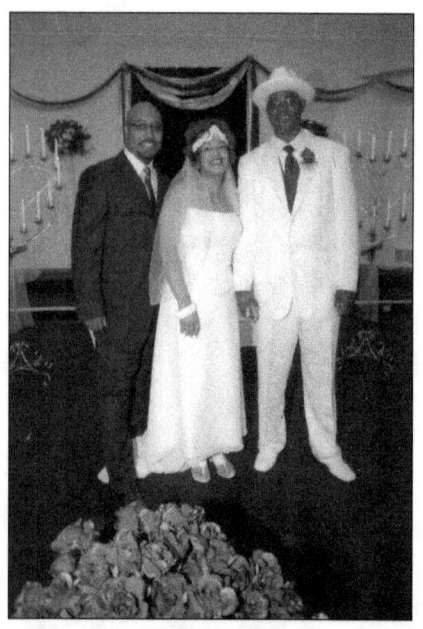

Left: Calvin and I pose with Bishop Hugh Smith Jr., the Pastor of Emmanuel Covenant Church International in Battle Creek. Michigan; below: My stepmother Ethel Mann; below, Bishop Smith with Pastor J.C. Oliver; below left, from left: Tracey Hodges, Shawna Earl, and Aunt Judith Tyler (Calvin's aunt), pose with me during our big day.

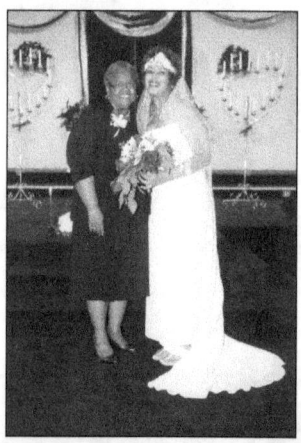

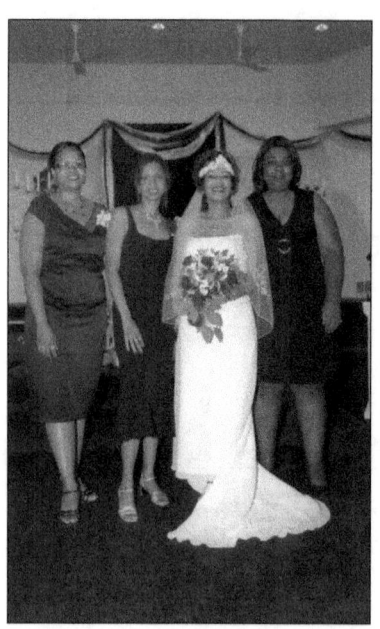

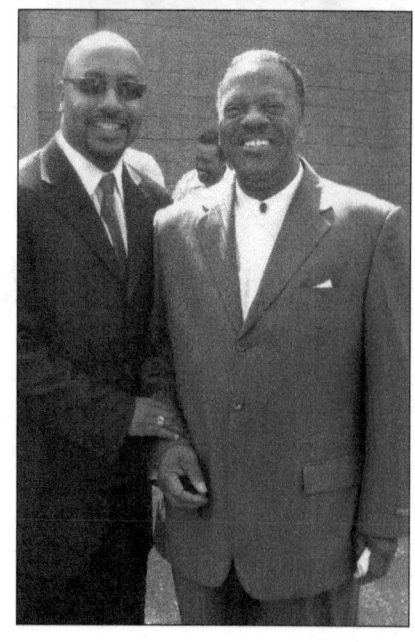

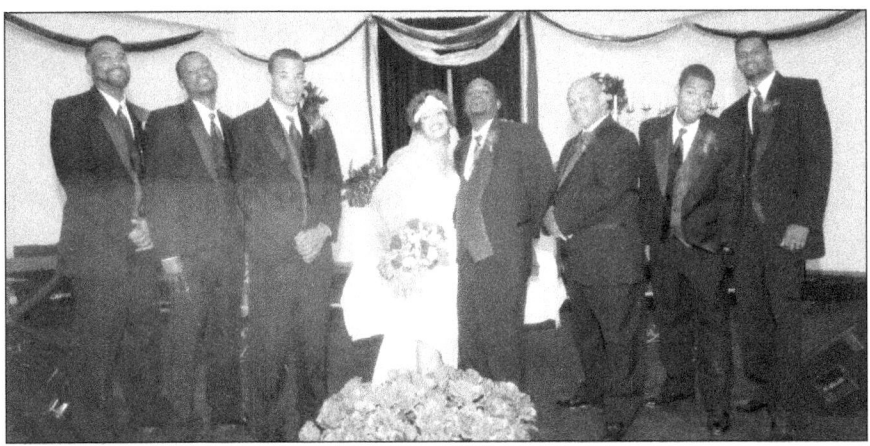

Above: The best man and groomsmen made my day even more special.

Below: The women in my wedding party included: Michelle Franklin, Esther Harden, Nicole Mann, Meria Wyrick-Colen, Me, Ola Hughes, Channel Wyrick, Charmia Wyrick, and Kathy McKinney-Mabry.

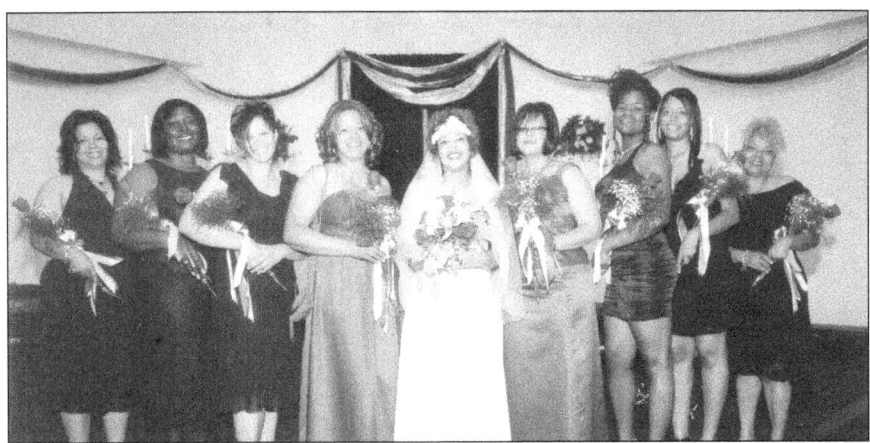

SMILE

In the mist of all my troubles,
Wondering if I have something good along
the way to smile about.

You woke me up this morning cheerful, sunny and bright to see
another lovely day.

You still love me enough to forgive me.

When I look up towards heaven and everything else that you have
created here on earth, I think of you.

This is my gift of joy I share with you.

A happy heart, a healing heart and a loving heart will help you get
through any test of storms in life.

If you didn't know, it's the Jesus that lives inside of me; that move me to
smile.

Now, I have something exciting to smile about,
because it all begins with you first, Lord.

When was the last time you show a smile?

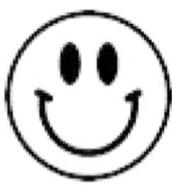

AFTERWORD

To make it simple and plain, Jesus is the Author and Finisher of my life. HE has blessed me with many unique gifts and talents in writing poetry and stories. My spirit motivates and inspires me to share with all people, God's love straight from the heart, which has been express to me through my loving grandmothers. I treasure each moment of them by keeping their spirit and memories alive in me.

Here on this journey, I shared with you about my healing, prayers, faith, relationships, and my miracle in 2007. Believe the unbelievable and receive the impossible.

In 2006, I celebrated my 50th birthday when I was seriously ill. Now, in 2017 (the year of this publication), I will be celebrating my 61st birthday healed and healthy in Jesus' Name.

In July 18, 2017, I celebrated the 10-year anniversary of my liver transplant. Hallelujah!

> *Delight thyself also in the Lord; and he shall*
> *give thee the desires of thine heart.*
> Psalm 37:4

THE VIRTUOUS WOMAN THAT I AM

In the beginning, God created a woman that one day would be suitable for a man named Adam from his rib. A woman named Eve, became his companion. "Then the Lord God said, It is not good that the man be alone. I will make a helper suitable for him" (Genesis 2:18).

God had spoken to Adam and Eve about a particular tree with fruit. This one was forbidden to eat from. God saw that Adam and Eve had hidden from his presence because of the sin that was brought onto them when they disobeyed God's words. God was disappointed.

Later, generations passed, but men seemed to still blame any woman for Eve's mistake. God soon got tired of seeing men and women corrupted in sin. God realized that it was time to make another plan, by sending His son Jesus, to save this world from the sins of both men and women.

"The laws of fruit of the spirit are love, joy, peace, long-suffering, gentleness, goodness, and faith" (Galatians 5:22). "Who can find a virtuous woman? for her price is far above rubies" (Proverb 31:10). She gave her heart and soul to become a spiritual woman. You cannot put a price on a virtuous woman; she is a true blessing from the Lord. "She will do him good not evil all the days of her life" (Proverbs 31:12).

To successfully exceed in any task or challenges in life, she will have to put on the armor of faith to go through the trials of tribulation. This will show the world she was chosen to become the virtuous woman that she is from God.

For the woman that I am, beautiful, strong, and bold, no matter if I am tall, short, rich or poor. The letter 'A' can say that I have a new Attitude that shows dignity in my walk and talk with God. She speaks truth and love that comes from her heart and spirit. No evil shall come from her tongue, but bring forth a holy smile, a shower of joy, and laughter to everyone's heart; I am a virtuous woman, that I am.

For the woman that I am, my body language will tell it all. Look at me, I am confident in my size and shape. So when I do step out in colorful fashion and style, it will reflect the richness and elegance that fit the clothes I wear. I am a virtuous woman, that I am.

Her natural beauty enhances the inner beauty of excellence that comes from Christ, so that her loveliness will flow in the Holy Spirit that has been anointed in her. Her outward beauty shines from within so that the make-up that she wears will not only be a reflection of radiance that glows upon her face but a virtuous woman, that I am.

The woman that I am, 'a message to men only.' As you walk past wondering what type of fragrance is in the midst of a breeze, don't inhale but exhale my, Chanel Coco Mademoiselle Perfume. You can't touch this, I'm a virtuous woman, that I am.

For the woman that I am, spirit of character and uniqueness; it begins with respect, relationships, walking in faith according to God's fruitful word filled with a loving spirit, standing on humility, boldness, believe in her responsibility, truthful, faithful, trustworthy, humorous, reliable, caring and express unconditional love In Jesus Name. I'm a virtuous woman, that I am.

Truly, there are virtuous women in my life. These women are living proof of a virtuous woman in 21st Century:

First Lady Letha Smith in Ann Arbor, MI; Co-Pastor Shannon Sweet in Battle Creek, MI; Dr. Janice Holmes-Mann in Detroit, MI; First Lady Sandy Graham in Battle Creek, MI; Mary Mann in Albion, MI; Ethel Mann in Battle Creek, MI; Edith Harvey in Atlanta, GA; Aunt Merie Archie in Battle Creek, MI; Aunt Violet Kelly in Detroit, MI; Judith Jones in Battle Creek, MI; Georgia Howard in Battle Creek, MI; Cherrie Williams in Battle Creek, MI; Betty Newsome in Kalamazoo, MI; Evelyn Miller in Kalamazoo, MI; Hazel Brown in Battle Creek, MI; Mrs. Doris Dearring in Detroit, MI; Mrs. Gloria Dearring in Battle Creek, MI; Lisa Henry in Battle Creek, MI; Patricia Gabriel in Battle Creek, MI; Jeanette Broadway (Nippy) in Battle Creek, MI; Pastor Donna Simmon in Battle Creek, MI; Esther Harden in Washington, DC; Michelle Franklin in Battle Creek, MI; Paula Stein in Battle Creek, MI; TeYonna Henry in Battle Creek, MI; Brady Patrick in Battle Creek, MI; Rhonda Whitlock in Battle Creek, MI; Kristena Drain-Williams in Battle Creek, MI; Charlene Drain in Battle Creek, MI; Felicia Williams in Battle Creek, MI; Katie Barnes in Battle Creek, MI; Yolydia Gray in Battle Creek, MI; Ethel Fitzpatrick in Battle Creek, MI; Marilyn Morris in Battle Creek, MI; Jeanette Payne in Lansing, MI; Carolyn Walker in Battle Creek, MI; Joyce Glass in Battle Creek, MI; Grace Cowens in Battle Creek, MI; Diane King in Battle Creek, MI, and Aunt Mary Smith in Thompson, GA. In addition, my beloved grandmothers, Arzola Edwards and Lizzie Mann rest in heavenly peace.

A story I wrote based on scriptures from Genesis and Proverbs.

LOVE LETTER DEDICATION

This book is first, dedicated to my Heavenly Father. I couldn't have made it without you! Words cannot ever paint a picture of love that I have for you.

I have been blessed and grateful to have a wonderful spiritual man of God, an anointed, humble counselor, truth-speaking man to guide me in God's Word, Bishop Hugh D. Smith Jr. He speaks honesty and helps me recognize my purposes in the Kingdom of God. He believes in healing and miracles, and his sweet wife Letha is a blessing. They dedicate their lives to serving the people of God. I thank them for being in my corner of healing. You two are truly angels sent from heaven on earth. I am thankful that God has placed you all in my heart, forever. I love you dearly in Jesus Name.

To Dr. Senior Pastor Frederick J. Sweet, a Godly man, a praying man of God, who truly loves the Lord and his lovely partner, Co-Pastor Shannon Sweet. Together I call them the dynamic duos of prayer, anointed man and woman in Christ Jesus. They always on fire ready to save souls and to serve God's purposes at Emmanuel Covenant Church International. When God chose Pastor Sweet to Pastor at the church. God and Bishop knew you were ordained to do an excellent job as our new Shepherd. I thank God for speaking HIS spirit in Pastor Sweet, to push me to finish my book by giving God all the glory, because it is not all about me, it's about HIM. I love you very much Senior Pastor Sweet in Jesus' Name.

To Co-Pastor Shannon Sweet, if it wasn't for your wisdom the title of my book, "There's Something Behind That Smile," probably wouldn't have exist if by chance I hadn't attended the wedding of Tiffany C. Hardeman-Moore and Antonio D. Kirk. Again, if by chance I had not stopped at the table to fellowship with you, Tena Moss and Sherrill Cotton-Smith. When Co-Pastor asked, "How was I coming along with my book? I still was trying to come up with a different title name. You said, "Sister Dot, you always smiling. That would make people wonder about the title and the story behind it, because that is what you do—you smile!" Everyone at the table agreed, they liked it too! Thanks again Co-Pastor, for helping me name my book. I dedicated this book to you, love you, your sunshine, Dot.

To my sweet, wonderful mother, Ola B. Mann, and my loving and understanding father, Willie Mann Jr., and my loving spiritual stepmother Ethel and stepsisters Stacey and Shauna, "Much love to you all, forever." To my lovely daughter, Nicole and to my remarkable, extraordinary, beautiful grandchildren, Jasmine Warren, Juan Warren II and Joshua Mann— "I'm so proud of you all, each one of you have been truly a blessing in grandmother's life!" I love you so much in Jesus' Name.

To Bishop Tino Smith and family; you all have shown me so much love over the years. Congratulations, again on your new book, "The Reproach Is Lifted." Thanks for all the love!

To Pastor Donna Simmons, thanks for help getting the Clubhouse to celebrate my dad's seventy-five birthday. This was his first and only birthday party he ever had. You are an angel! God Bless you beautiful!

To my fabulous sisters Ola Hughes, Judy Mann and brothers Bryant Mann and Darrick Mann. Darrick once again thanks for coming to Daddy's, seventy-fifth birthday; it truly made his day and he will never forget it. I will keep praying for my family, that one day, they will accept the Lord as their personal savior, in Jesus' Name. Love you all!

To Calvin Wyrick, my heavenly sent, strong, hard-working, and handsome husband. "Only you can make me happy." Love you very much, honey, in Jesus' Name!

To my lovely sister-in-law, Meria Wyrick, keep singing like an angel unto the Lord with all your heart. God's love is going to bless you so dearly. You are on your journey to stardom and prosperity. Keep up the good work in Jesus Name. Love ya!

To my three gorgeous, sweet nieces, Anquette Henderson, who was there when I needed your help in cleaning my house and applying ointment on me; Kelsie Mann, and Stephanie King—we need to keep in touch more! I will always love you all in Jesus' Name.

To my only fine nephew, Christopher King a genuine, good-hearted young man who has nothing but love for me! Congratulations, on the new arrival of your baby boy! I have nothing but love for you nephew.

To a sweet stepdaughter, Leondriss C. Wyrick, enjoy driving your new automobile and my handsome stepson Marquis Jackson who loves eating my cupcakes. I love you both forever in Jesus' Name.

To my loving first cousins, Dr Janice Holmes, her husband Pastor Bennie Holmes and your three lovely children you all mean the world to me. We always believe in keeping in contact with one another, our relationships as cousins has been nothing but love and kindness straight from the heart. We love Jesus! I am very blessed to have beautiful cousins in Atlanta, Georgia, Edith Harvey, Michael Harvey, Geoffrey Harvey, Gemahri Harvey; My good looking cousins in Thompson, GA, Daniel Mann, David Mann, Jr, James Mann, Robert "Pat" Smith, Willie "Rooster" Henry Smith, Jr, Darryl L. Smith, Phillip Smith, John H. Smith and Ronnie Woodard.

To my loving cousins here in Michigan, Hertis Mann, Ericka Mann, Elder Edmon and Mary Mann who I enjoy traveling to Detroit; My loveable aunt Jackie Edwards, Larry Edwards, Lonnie Edwards, Michael Edwards, Pat Edwards, Wilma Edwards, Butchie Edwards, Tammy Edwards, Janie Edwards, Freddie Perry, Little Willie Edwards, Zanudra Perry and NicHole Milton and family. Love you all my adorable cousins in Jesus' Name!

To my loving mother-in-law, Doris Dearring whose word is, "believe that every woman needs to be treated as a Queen, to be beautiful, strong, used wisdom and have confident in yourself." Love you mom, for all that you have done for me in the past. You will always be my inspiration, spiritual mother-in-law. My heart to yours, love you all! To my loving sister-in-laws the Dearring women: Deborah, Trivia, and Yvette. To my brother-in-laws, Dewayne, Brian, and my ex-husband, What a blessing to have you all in my life. Thank you for accepting me for who I am. Much love in Jesus' Name.

To my Dearring family in Battle Creek, my beautiful, aunt Gloria, your two sweet, loving daughters, Shellie and Deborah, nothing but love for me! Your son, Charles continues getting your education. Thanks, for caring and being a part of my life. Love you!

To my two dearest, oldest, best girls, Michelle Franklin and Esther Harden. It seems like it was only yesterday and we are still best of friends in 2016. When God put you both in my path as my fabulous sista's for a reason and a season, forever. I am truly, truly blessed to have a spiritual relationship with two beautiful real friends. I love you both so much in Jesus' Name!

What a blessing to have dear friends in my life. You all cared about me from the beginning of the journey. Even when I was going through my ills, you all were there to help. Some of us have been friends for many years, and it has been a pleasure to have among loving friends with a heart, forever. May God bless each one of you with good health and prosperity in Jesus' Name!

To my glamorous sister-girls, Jeanette Broadway (Nippy), Katie Barnes, Pat Doggett, Jeanette Payne, Kathy Mabry, Marilyn Morris, Mary Cusic, Jewell Thomas, Linda Burnside and Victoria Tibbs. God allow us to come together on his path so that one day we can be a blessing to one another in our lives. Who said that too many women could not get along? I believe someone lied! Love you all forever in Jesus' Name.

To my two lovely princess my godchildren, Bianca and Aja Smith; you are beautiful and blessed to have an understanding and caring mother, Michelle. Love you so much! You will always be in my heart. I have not forgotten you in Jesus' Name.

To my lovely, sweet, and praying aunt Violet Kelly, who lives in Detroit, who I love you very much! We enjoy talking about the Lord, every time on the phone each day. I have nothing but love, aunt Violet in Jesus' Name.

My dearest and beautiful, aunt Mary Smith that lives in Thomaston, GA, who turn 93 years old on September 8, 2017—when the doctors said she wasn't going to live passed the age of thirty-six years old because she had polio in her right leg. Look at God! You are still here living and looking good. Love you auntie in Jesus Name.

To my families, relatives, dearest friends and Federal Center coworkers, spiritual sisters and brothers that is in my life, now! I thank God for having a real genuine relationship and love for me in this world. God knew actually the right people to put in my path. What an incredible place to have a job with people that had a loving heart. I miss you all so much. I hope to see you all at my book signing!

To all my other loving friends, spiritual mothers, thank you for being a part of my life, a seasonal friendship, and you will be forever in my heart, love you all, such as: Vee Williams, April Matthews, Rhonda Hoag, Val Mabry, Felicia Williams, Vanessa Tucker, Kristina Drain, Charlene Drain, Sherrill Smith-Cotton, Yolydia & Ben Gray. Angela J. Johnson-Patton, Loretta Willis, Ashley Smith, Gila Williams, Reba Bolden, Lisa and Larry Henry, Ethel and Keith Fitzpatrick, Rosia Howard, Hazel Brown, Doris Jones, Judith and Roosevelt Jones, Roberta Cribbs, Georgia Howard, Evelyn Miller, Betty Newman, Mother Hardeman and Father Hardeman, Cherrie Williams, Grace Washington, Magie Irby, Patricia Gariel, Mother Nell Rosa, and Joyce Eldred who hired me at the Federal Center and many more loving friends that I will always treasure in my heart forever, in Jesus' Name!

Dear God, thank you for the anointed man and woman, Pastor Graham and First Lady Sandy Graham, you both have been a true blessing to me, knowing you in this life though Calvin. You both are real! Let us try to get together a little more often this year, because it is good to be around good people that love the Lord. Calvin and I have nothing but love for the two of you in Jesus' Name! "Preach the word!"

In 2017 I had worked at Macy's for eight years as a sales associate in Battle Creek, MI and I love it! I have to thank Laura who hired me to work as a flextime associate in the fragrances department. I was blessed to have a delightful and positive supervisor named Mark. My store manager's name was Mary, who had a genuine warm and loving spirited at heart (I missed you both).

My girl, Tracy you rock. Brenda, love your beautiful sense of humor, and Abbey, "What's up my sista?" In addition, I have to give a shout out to my lovely, adorable, fabulous former sales associate that rock, Michelle, Pam, Dawn, Vincent, JoAnn, and Barbara whom I have worked with the longest. To the other gorgeous sales associates that rock, who I enjoy working with daily, Alayzia Acacia, Alicia, Laura Taylor, Whitney Akers, Vanessa, Brooke Massa, and Leslee Popovich-Smith. Love Ya, in Jesus' Name.

There were other sales associates who I worked with in the past, Denisha Sanders, Carolyn Cheek, Sara, Trisha, Kim Parker, Julie, Theresa, Delta, Lisa, and many more in the other departments, Valerie Jones, Nancy, Pam, Lisa, Morgan, Rebecca, Sierra, Carol and Trish. To all my Macy's customers, You're the best! Love you all! I love working with all my Macy's sale's associates and Macy's customers. God bless you all!

I would sincerely like to thank James Smith, for taking the time out of your busy schedule to introduce me to Sean and Sonya Hollins, who are my publishing consultants. Congratulations, on your oncoming inspirational book in the near future. I know you will have many more delightful stories to write for all the people to read. God bless you! James, you and Senior Pastor Frederick J. Sweet inspired me to step out of my comfort zone to get my story published. I thank you, beautiful Laura Taylor, and Meria Wyrick, for helping me revised my proof book. You all are my angels. God bless you, and I love you, in Jesus' Name.

HISTORY

"Transplantation: Where It's Been, Where It's Going,"
The following was taken from a book called A Patient's Guide to Transplantation written by John P. Butorac & Mary M. Palancher

Far back in history (and mythology), there have been accounts of transplanting organs and body parts. The first reported heart transplant was performed by Pien Csiao and Hua To in China about 200BC according to legend. The Third Century Christian saints Cosmos and Damian earned their glory in part because of their reported leg transplantation.

However, it was not until the 18th century that researchers really began experimenting with organ transplantation in animals and humans. Obviously, these early scientists experienced many failures. But by the mid Twentieth Century, successful organ transplants became possible.

TRANSPLANT MILESTONES

1682 – First bone transplant, using a piece of skull from a dog;

1881 – First skin transplant;

1906 – First cornea transplant;

1906 – First successful knee joint transplant;

1906 – First kidney transplants, from sheep, pigs, goats and primates with no anti-rejection drugs;

1936 – First human to human kidney transplant Dr. Voronoy, Russia;

1943 – Development of dialysis machine;

1934 – Discovery that rejection is based on immunological factors Sir Peter Medawar, England;

1950 – First kidney transplant Dr. Richard Lawler, Little Mary Hospital Chicago, Illinois;

1954 – First successful kidney transplant living donor Dr. Jospeh E. Murray, Brigham and Women's Hospital, Boston Massachusetts;

1956 – First heart valve transplant;

1962 – Introduction of Imuran (azathioprine);

1962 – First successful kidney transplant, cadaver donor Peter BAENT Brigham Hospital, Boston, Massachusetts;

1963 – First human liver transplant Dr. Thomas E. Starzl, University of Colorado Medical School, Denver, Colorado;

1963 – First lung transplant Dr. James D. Hardy, University of Mississippi in Jackson, Mississippi;

1966 – First successful pancreas transplant Dr. William Kelly and Richard Lillehei, University of Minnesota, Minneapolis, Minnesota;

1967 – First heat transplant Dr.Christiaan Barnard, Groote Shuur Hospital, Capetown, South Africa;

1968 – First successful heart transplant Dr. Norman Shumway, Stanford University Hospital, Stanford, California;

1978 – Discovery of cyclosporine Jean Borel, Switzerland;

1979 – First U.S. clinical trials of Sandimmune (cyclosporine) in cadaver kidney transplants Peter Bent Brigham Hospital, Boston, Massachusetts, University of Colorado, Denver, Colorado;

1981 – First successful heart-lung transplant Dr. Bruce Reitz, Stanford University Hospital, Stanford, California;

1983 - U.S. Federal Drug Administration approves Sandimmnune (cyclosporine) for kidney, liver, and heart transplants;

1983 – First successful single lung transplant Dr. Joel Cooper, Toronto General Hospital, Toronto, Ontario, Canada;

1985 – First successful use of an artificial heart implant as a "bridge" to transplant University of Arizona, Tucson, Arizona;

1986 – Introduction of monoclonal antibodies into clinical medicine (OKT3) Dr. A. Benedict Cosimi, Massachusetts General Hospital, Boston, Massachusetts;

1986 – First successful double lung transplant Dr. Joel Cooper, Toronto General Hospital, Toronto, Ontario, Canada;

1987 – First successful liver-intestine transplant London, Ontario, Canada;

1988 - First split liver transplant with two recipients Paul Brousse Hospital, Villejuif, France;

1989 – First living liver donor transplant Sao Paulo, Brazil;

1989 – First successful living-related liver transplant Dr. Christopher Broelsch, University of Chicago Medical Center, Chicago, Illinois;

1989 – U.S. Federal Drug Administration approves Prograf (FK56) for transplants;

1990 – First successful living related lung transplant Dr. Vaughn A. Starnes, Stanford University Medical Center, Stanford, California;

1990 – U.S. Federal Drug Administration approves CellCept (mycophenolate mofetil);

1995 – U.S. Federal Drug Administration approves Neoral (new formulation of cyclosporine)

1996 – First laparoscopic live-donor nephrectomy Dr. Lloyd Ratner and Dr. Louis Kavoussi, John Hopkins Bayview Medical Center, Baltimore, Maryland;

1998 – First hand transplant Edward Herriott Hospital, Lyon, France;

1999 – First U.S. hand transplant Jewish Hospital, Louisville, Kentucky.

Notes: On Early Stages of Primary Biliary Cirrhosis (PBC)

James Neuberger, Consultant Physician, Queen Elizabeth Hospital's

Notes: On Early Stages of Primary Biliary Cirrhosis (PBC)

From the point of view of the medical profession, a person having an uncommon disease such as Primary Biliary Cirrhosis (PBC) has both disadvantages and advantages. It has disadvantages in, very often, the family doctor will not have looked after patients with PBC before and, therefore, may be unaware of many of the symptoms, signs and therapies available.

On the converse side, once the disease is diagnosed, doctors are very keen to learn more about the disease and will very often treat the per-

son as 'special.' Perhaps the biggest problem in early PBC is that the person looks extremely well. The slight pigmentation of the skin that is very often present, together with a tingle of jaundice, often makes the individual look as though she has just come back from
a visit to the Bahamas.

Yet it is very clear that outward appearances often believe what is going on inside. The tiredness which is associated with PBC appears to be totally different from any other sort of tiredness. It is not the same as when you have had a late night and all one can do is just advice the person to 'roll with the punches.'

At the moment there is extremely little research going on into the cause and treatment of the tiredness. It is not due to depression. Mark Swain in Canada has undertaken some recent work suggesting that there may be an abnormality of the axis between the pituitary and the adrenal glands.

Although many groups are working hard to find a cause for PBC, relatively few are trying to find out why people get so tired. Sympathy from the family doctor, from the hospital and above all from family and friends is the best therapy, but clearly does little to make a difficult situation bearable.

It must be remembered that liver function tests bear no guide to the severity of the lethargy and is also important to remember that the lethargy is often cyclical in nature, lasting maybe for two to three months, before resolving for a while.

It is important, however, that treatable causes of lethargy are considered: conditions such as poorly functioning thyroid gland, or the effect of medication, may sometimes cause a fall of tiredness. Of course, some patients with PBC do have depression. This usually causes symptoms distinct from the lethargy and responds well to therapy, which may be counseling, or medication for a while.

The other symptom of PBC is itching. Not everybody with itching has PBC and not everybody with PBC has itching. (Unfortunately, I received itching with the PBC; no medication would stop the itching. Also, I had tried all types of creams in the store over the counter and prescription cream for itching, the only treatment to stop the itching was to have a liver transplantation.

I was not aware how serious my condition was or chose to educate myself on how to receive a transplant if one was needed. I did not believe that transplants could happen in our culture. Most of the times we usually destroy the liver by bring harmful to it. Because of the rarity of PBC, many patients suffer for weeks or months the nature of the itching defined.

Doctors have stories of patients who have been referred, even to psychiatrists, before the diagnosis is eventually made. The doctor who I am referring to is, Lord who I only trust in. Yes, doctors had to evaluate me to see where my mind was at; but the power of prayer and God's Word was all I needed in the world. Thank you, Lord for the blood! That is what kept me from losing my mind; believing and trusting HIM in my heart).

You must remember that there are many causes of itching and PBC is a rare one. Nonetheless, when itching is due to PBC, there are potential therapies available. There is no doubt that Questran, or Questran light is highly effective and provided the patient can tolerate enough of it for long enough, then the vast majority of itching will be brought under control. There are a number of other alternative therapies, which can be used. It is extremely rare for the ultimate therapy, namely transplantation, to be used for extreme itching.

Again, we do not really understand the pathogenesis of itching in PBC. Older reports that it was due to bile acid appears to be wrong and more recent research has concentrated on naturally occurring opiate-like drugs. Those of you who have read, "Thomas de Quincey's Confessions of an English Opium Eater" will know that the opium addict did suffer, on occasion, from intractable itching. There are naturally occurring opiate-like substances produced naturally within the body and nothing to do with drugs–illicit or other! and it is through these may be involved in itching of PBC.

Finally, do remember that other symptoms and problems occur in people with PBC, even at an early stage. Aches and pains in bones, muscles and joints are not uncommon. Do check things over with your doctor, it may be that the symptoms are just a manifestation of the disease, but sometimes other causes are involved. Just because you have PBC it does not stop you from getting other problems.

It must be remembered that, with all people, with relatively rare diseases, the doctor might well be slow in reaching a diagnosis and once the diagnosis is reached, may well require further information to have up-to-date information about the condition. It is, therefore, particularly important to have available not only an organization, such as the PBC Foundation, to provide information both for medical staff and paramedical staff, but also an organization that will give people help with the disease all the information they require and where necessary the option to share it with fellow sufferers according to James Neuberger, Consultant Physician, Queen Elizabeth Hospital, Birmingham.

*This is based on work in rats, but how far results in rats can be extrapolated to humans with PBC remains uncertain.

Primary Biliary Cirrhosis (PBC)

Those who suffer from PBC, and their families, may say one day, "Oh, Lord, whoever finds a cure for itching will be making a fortune!" Unfortunately, we can only hope, pray, keep the faith and press toward the mark for the prize of the High calling of God in Christ Jesus. (Philippians 3:14). Here are a few hints that helped me make it through the itching below:

- Always keep your nails cut short to avoid scratching your skin.
- Avoid very hot baths or being over-heated in bed.
- Do not wear nylon or wool next to your skin – cotton is best. In the summer, the ultra-violet rays in the sun can help, but please remember to take the usual precautions when out in the sun, to avoid burning.
- Try a teacup full of bicarbonate soda in a cool bath. Soak up to the neck for approximately twenty minutes. It is particularly helpful.
- Just before going to bed, if your scalp is itchy, rinse in water containing bicarbonate of soda after washing it. If the soles your feet are itchy, soak them in a basin of water with bicarbonate of soda.
- If you have taken Questran sachets, please make sure you drink it before or during your meal and not after the meal. Take the Questran before breakfast, lunch and tea. It a waste of time to take it at bedtime when you are not eating. If you do not like the taste, try adding squash.
- Do not use perfumed soap, bath essence, shower gel, or talcum powder.
- Finally, please always tell your doctor about your itching. They may have a prescription to suggest that you have not tried be fore. For those of you who do not have any itch, it does not mean it will happen in the future. Some patients never itch!

GLOSSARY

From "A Patient's Guide to Transplantation" by John P. Butorac & Mary M. Palanchar

Acute: having severe symptoms and a short course.

Acute Rejection: the body's attempt to destroy a transplanted organ–usually occurs within the first year after transplant.

Adverse Reaction: see Side Effect.

Allocation: the system of distributing donated organs and tissues to patients in need of a transplant.

Allograph: an organ that is removed from a donor to be used in another person.

Anemia: a condition characterized by too few red blood cells in the bloodstream, resulting in insufficient oxygen to tissues and organs.

Antibody: a protein that is produced by the body's immune system when it detects a foreign substance, such as a transplanted organ.

Antibiotic: a drug used to fight bacterial infections.

Antigen: a substance, such as a transplanted organ, that can trigger an immune response. The immune response may be the production of antibodies.

Anti-Rejection Drug: see Immunosuppressant

Arteriogram: an X-ray of the arteries taken with the aid of a dye, sometimes referred to as angiography.

Ascites: accumulation of fluid in the stomach, usually associated with liver disease.

AST: acronym for the American Society of Transplantation (formerly the American Society of Transplant Physicians).

ASTS: acronym for the American Society of Transplant Surgeons.

Bacteria: microscopic organisms that invade human cells multiply rapidly and produce toxins that interfere with normal cell functions.

Beta Blockers: a class of drugs that lower blood pressure.

Bile: fluid produced by the liver that is transported to the intestines to help digestion and remove waste products.

Bile Ducts: passage ways in and from the liver that transport bile.

Bilirubin: a substance in bile that is produced when the liver processes waste products. A high bilirubin level causes yellowing of the skin.

Biliary Cirrhosis: slow, progressive scarring of the bile ducts in the liver.

Biopsy: removal of tissue for examination under a microscope.

Bone Marrow: spongy tissue in the cavities of large bones, where blood cells are produced.

Brain Death: the condition when the brain has creased functioning, as determined by the medical team. Cadaveric organs usually are recovered from persons declared brain dead.

Cadaveric Organ: an organ from a person who has been declared brain dead.

Candidate: a person who is waiting for a transplant.

Cardiac: relating to the heart.

Catheter: a small, flexible plastic tube inserted into the body to administer or remove fluids.

Chronic: persisting for a long time.

Chronic Rejection: slow failure of transplanted organ.

Cirrhosis: irreversible scarring of the liver. Can be caused be a variety of conditions.

Coagulation: relating to the process of clotting, usually the body's system of controlling bleeding.

Compliance: the process of a patient following the instructions of his transplant center, especially regarding his medication regimen.

Cornea: the transparent outer coat of the eyeball. Corneas can be donated and transplanted.

Corticosteroid: see Steroid.

Crossmatch: a test for recipient antibodies versus donor antigens. A positive crossmatch means the recipient and donor are incompatible. Crossmatching is routinely done for kidney and pancreas patients.

Cyclosporine: a drug commonly used after organ transplantation to suppress the immune system of the recipient and prevent rejection of the transplanted organ by the immune system.

Dialysis: a mechanical process of cleaning the blood of patients with kidney failure.

Diastolic: the bottom number of a blood pressure reading measuring the heart at rest.

Distension: a visible protrusion of the abodomen.

Diuresis: significantly increasing the production of urine.

Department of Transplantation (DOT): the office of the federal government whose principal responsibilities include management of the Organ Procurement and Transplantation Network (OPTN), the Scientific Registry of Transplant Recipients (SRTR) and the National Marrow Donor Program (NMDP).

Donor: someone from whom an organ or tissue is used for transplantation.

Donor Card: a card that states a person's wishes to be an organ and or tissue donor.

Edema: abnormal accumulation of fluid in the body which causes swelling.

Encephalopathy: confused, fuzzy or slowed thinking when the liver is not functioning properly. At its extreme, it can result in coma.

End Stage Organ Disease: a disease that leads to permanent failure of an organ.

End Stage Renal Disease (ESRD): failure of the kidneys requiring the patient to need dialysis or kidney transplant for survival.

Fulminant: happening very quickly and severely.

Gallbladder: a small pocket that stores bile.

Gastrointestinal: relating to the stomach and intestines.

Genetic Matching: see Tissue Typing.

Gingival Hypertrophy: enlargement of the gums as a side effect of certain medications, especially cyclosporine.

Glucose: a type of sugar in the blood.

Graft: a transplanted tissue or organ.

Harvest: a term, often offensive to donor families, used to describe retrieval of a donor organ. See Recovery.

HCFA: acronym for the United States Health Care Finance Administration. HCFA provides funding for federal health care related programs, such as Medicare.

Health and Human Service (HHS): the department of the federal government who is responsible for health- related programs and issues.

Heart: the organ that pumps blood received from the veins into the arteries, thereby supplying the entire circulatory system.

Hemorrhage: excessive bleeding.

Hepatic: relating to the liver.

HHS: see Health and Human Services.

High Blood Pressure: a condition where the force of the blood pushing against the walls of the blood vessels in higher than normal.

Hirsutism: excessive increase in hair growth.

HLA: Human Leukocyte Antigens. Molecules found on cell in the body that characterizes each person as unique. In donor-recipient matching, HLA determines the organs match.

Hypertension: see High Blood Pressure.

Immune System: the body's nature defense mechanism against invasion by foreign bodies. In transplantation, the transplanted organ is considered a foreign body and the recipient's immune system will naturally want to defend against it through rejection of the organ.

Immunosuppressant: a drug that is taken to help the body accept a transplanted organ by suppressing the immune system.

Immunosuppression: the artificial suppression of the immune response, usually through drugs, so that the body will not reject a transplanted organ or tissue.

Intestine: the portion of the digestive system extending from the stomach to the anus.

Intravenous: into a vein – usually refers to medication of fluid that is infused into a vein through a catheter.

Jaundice: yellowing of the skin and eyes. A sign that the liver or bile Duct system is not working normally.

Kidney: one of a pair of organs that remove waste from the body through the production of urine.

Liver: the largest internal organ. The liver removes toxic substances from the blood, secretes bile into the bowel to aid in digestion, and helps process proteins, carbohydrates, and fats, among other vital functions.

Lung: one of a pair of respiratory organs functioning to supply oxygens to the blood and remove carbon dioxide.

Multiple Listing: being on the waiting list at more than one transplant center.

Noncompliance: failure of a patient to following the instructions of His transplant center, especially regarding his medication regimen.

National Organ Transplant Act (NOTA): the law passed by Congress in 1984, which outlawed the sale of human organs and initiated the development of a national systems for organ sharing and a scientific registry to collect and report transplant data.

Organ Procurement and Transplant Network (OPTN): the nationwide network responsible for organ procurement, allocation and distribution. The OPTN consists of UNOS and many OPOs throughout the United States.

Organ Procurement Organization (OPO): a local organization that coordinates organ procurement (retrieval, or recovery) activities within a designated area. OPO activities include evaluating potential donors, discussing donation with surviving family members, arranging for surgical removal and transport of donated organs and educating the public about the need for donation.

Pancreas: the long, irregularly shaped gland which secrets pancreatic fluid into the lower end of the stomach to aid in the digestion of proteins, carbohydrates and fats.

Platelets: the smallest elements in the blood – needed to control bleeding.

Preservation: special methods of keeping a donated organ viable between procurement and transplantation.

Procurement: see Recovery.

Prognosis: the predicated or likely outcome.

Protocol: the plan of treatment.

Pulmonary: relating to the lungs.

Recipient: a person who has received a transplant.

Recovery: the removal or retrieval of organs and tissues for transplantation.

Rejection: an event when the immune system tries to fight off a transplanted organ.

Renal: relating to the kidneys.

Transplantation: the transplantation of a new organ after the rejection or failure of a previously transplanted organ.

Scientific Registry of Transplant Recipients (SRTR): the organization that collects and reports data on transplant recipients.

Sensitization: the condition where a potential recipient has antibodies in his blood that make cross-matching less like – usually because of pregnancy, blood transfusion, or previous rejection of a transplanted organ.

Side Effect: an unintended (but not necessarily unexpected) reaction to a drug.

Small Bowel: see Intestine.

Status: a code used to indicate the relative degree of medical urgency for a patient waiting for a heart or liver transplant.

Steroid: one of a group of medications including Prednisone and Solu-Medrol.

Systolic: the top number of a blood pressure reading measuring the heart when it is contracting.

Thoracic: relating to the heart, lungs, and chest.

Tissue Typing: a blood test identifying a genetic marker. Tissue typing is done for all kidney donors' recipients to determine a proper match.

Transplantation, Allogeneic: see Allograph.

Transplantation, Autologous: transplantation of an organism's own cells or tissues back into itself.

Tranaplantation, Xenogenic: see Xenograph,

UNOS: United Network for Organ Sharing.

Varices: enlarged veins that can develop in the esophagus and stomach with liver disease.

Vascular: relating to blood vessels.

Xenograph: transplantation between members of a different species, e.g., the transplantation of animal organs into humans.

THE FUTURE

And where does transplantation go from here? There are the constant incremental improvements–improved surgical techniques, better medication management, etc., that result in improved survival rates and improved quality of life for patients. Almost daily, we read accounts of new breakthroughs, not only in scientific and medical journals, but also in the popular press.

There are:

- LVADS (heart assist machines):
- Surgical techniques that may eliminate the need for transplants for some heart patients;
- Liver "dialysis" machines that can take over failing liver function to 'buy time" for a patient waiting for a new liver;
- Split liver transplants so one liver can save two lives;
- Partial liver transplants, living liver donor transplants;
- Xenotransplants, growing genetically-altered animals to supply organs;
- Growing organs from stem cells in laboratories;
- Implanting liver cells that will replace a damaged liver; refurbishing old donor hearts that previously would have been discarded.
- And what about transplant patients?
- New drugs with fewer side effects?
- One-shot immunosuppression?
- Selective immunosuppression?

IN LOVING MEMORY

"Not a day goes by wishing you were all still here."

Alyce M. Woodard (aunt), August 7, 1918 – May 9, 1994.

Arzola Tipton-Edwards (maternal grandmother), September 9, 1910 – October 21, 1994.

Authar Mae Mann (aunt), unknown

Bertha Alexander (church member), August 12, 1929 – May 10, 1988.

Dan Edwards (paternal grandfather), unknown

Danny Edwards-Holmes (cousin), October 29, 1952 – April 1, 1994.

David P. Mann, Sr. (paternal uncle), June 9, 2005 – June 3, 2005.

Doris E. Dearring (mother-in-law) May 23, 1935 -September 28, 2017.

Drue Cilla Mann (aunt), July 29, 1928 – January 6, 2012.

Emma Elizabeth (Broughton) Ampey (friend), Sept. 29, 1924–Aug. 6, 2013.

Floyd L. McKinney (my daughter's dad), Dec. 15, 1955–Sept. 26, 2012.

Fred Gene Perry (cousin), April 4, 1948 – April 28, 2011.

Gene L. Hughes, Sr. (brother-in-law), Feb. 14, 1950 – Jan. 24, 2008.

Homer, Dearring, (uncle Charles), September 1, 1941 - May 21, 2009.

Hugh D. Smith, Sr. (my Bishop's father), Feb. 24, 1943–May 24, 2015.

Jackie D. Williams (church member), August 25, 1936 – May 14, 2007.

Jenny Vee Perry (cousin), August 2, 1949 – March 9, 1983.

Joseph C. Mann (paternal uncle), June 11, 1923 – April 14, 2005.

Larry LaShawn Crosswright (Nicole's brother), Nov. 13, 1972 -Nov. 4, 2012.

Latoya Te'Nae Cooper (brother-in-law's niece), April 6, 1983-November 10, 2015.

Leo Dell Perry, Jr. (church friend), June 12, 1939 - December 11, 2016

Linnie A. Prior (maternal great-grandmother) 1888 – March 1975.

Lizzie Mae Mann (paternal grandmother), July 7, 1903– April 20, 1995.

Londa L. Hunter-Walls (church member and friend), April 11, 1962–August 3, 2011.

Maggie Bolden Fortune (church member), Aug. 16, 1923–Nov. 6, 2013.

Marilyn Crawford (church member and friend), May 18, 1954–Oct. 31, 2009.

Michael D. Scott (church member and friend), Nov. 24, 1956–May 10, 2005.

Morris Mann (paternal uncle), Aug. 16, 1938–Dec. 24, 1999.

Oranganell Harbin (dear friend), September 11, 1958–April 27, 2014. (known as "Nell Harbin").

Pat Smith (cousin in Georgia), August 27, 1954 – March 20, 2012.

Patricia A. Edwards (cousin), October 21, 1950 – December 8, 2007.

Rosa L. Austin (Mother of the church and friend), March 22, 1920–July 18, 2001.

Tim Grier (My grandmother's sister), unknown

Timmie Edwards (maternal aunt), March 22, 1931–Aug. 9, 1995.

Vivian K. Pierce (church member), December 20, 1944–January 18, 2014, (known as "Mother Kay").

Willie Edwards (maternal uncle), Aug. 06, 1929–Feb. 2, 1999.

Willie H. Smith, Jr. (cousin in Georgia), November 16, 1949–Feb. 2, 2010. (known as "Rooster")

Willie Mann, Sr. (paternal grandfather), Feb. 2, 1897–April 4, 1984.

Willie Perry (cousin, (known as little "Willie"), unknown.

In loving memory of Doris Dearring - May 23, 1935 - Sep 28, 2017

CONCLUSION & ACKNOWLEDGEMENTS

I am very grateful to all who those who attended the wedding and gave generous blessings.

Bishop Hugh D. Smith, Jr., First Lady Letha, & Bethany Smith; Mrs. Doris Dearring, Trivia Dearring, Deborah Dearring and family; Hazel Brown and family; Ronnie & Michelle Franklin, Esther Harden, Loretta Whitt, Jeanette Payne, Pastor Elroy and Darlene Morris; Angela Johnson-Patton, Floyd & Ola Hughes, Linda Cooper, RaMyiah Renae Cooper, Annie Hughes, Fred Hughes and wife, Dorothy Hughes; William Tate, Pastor Bennie and Dr Janice Holmes, Philip Holmes, Georgia Howard, Ashley Smith, John & Mary Jackson; Gail and George (neighbors); Ethel Mann, Pastor Donna Simmons, Theresa & Bo Brooks; Grace Cowens, Liz Alexander & granddaughter, Debra Levy, Michael & Shawna Earl and family; Tracey Hodges, Edwards & Delores Hooks; Aunt Jacqueline Lathan, Wilma Edwards, Lonnie Edwards, Michael Edwards, Jamie Edwards, Aishi Willis and family; Roosevelt & Judith Jones; Ericka Mann, Elder Edmon & Mary Mann; Leon Wyrick and guests; Charles Colen, Charles Colen Jr., Raneko and family; Jeanette Broadway (Nippy), Sylvia Shelton and family; Tilar Hampton, Creighton Mabry, Cherrie Williams, Brian & Sherrill Cotton-Smith; Carolyn Walker, Leatrice Dunkin, Margie Irby, Mr. & Mrs. Dea Holmes; Java Holiday, Kathy Mabry, Larry & Edna Dorsey, Debbie & Anthony Buckney; Tommie & Margaret Kirk; Floyd & Kim Parker; Paula Stein, Senior Pastor Frederick & Copastor Shannon Sweet; Erica Mann, Kelise Mann, Anquette Henderson, Nicole Mann, Jasmine Warren, Juan Warren II, Joshua Mann, Bryant Mann, Ola Mann, Mattie Childs, Mary Cusic, Grace Washington, Alvin, Fred & Tina Trust; Bennie Drain, Kristina Drain, Charlene Drain, Grace Washington, Brandon Weddle, Charla Hinds, Artesia Hinds & family; Linda Burnside & mother; Matonya Wyrick, The Flower's Family, Lloyd & Lisa DeWalker and family; Mary Williams, Judith Taylor, Leondisa Wyrick, Channel Wyrick, Charmia Wyrick, Kathy Mabry, Christopher King, Marquis Jackson, Michael Hightower, and Freddie Perry. There were many friends sending us beautiful cards with a love blessing: Ted Hubbard, Aunt Gloria Dearring, Michelle Moore, Aunt Violet Kelly, Rose Miller & family; Victoria Tibbs, Jewell Thomas, Dorothy Peoples, Pam Swift, Auntie Merie Archie, Jean Lanier and Cathy Mabry.

ABOUT THE AUTHOR

Author Dorothy M. Wyrick is a native of Battle Creek, Michigan where she was born on August 19, 1956. She graduated from Battle Creek Central High School in 1974, and after the birth of her daughter, she began working at the Battle Creek Federal Center (1980-2007). She retired from the Federal Center due to her illness from the liver disease diagnosis in 2000.

Even though doctors were giving her a grim prognosis, she held on to her faith that God "had her back." She has been a member of Emmanuel Covenant Church International for twenty-eight years under the leadership of Founder Bishop Hugh D. Smith, Jr., currently led by Dr. Senior Pastor Frederick and Co-pastor Shannon L. Sweet.

There's Something Behind That Smile, shares of Dorothy's relationships, spiritual foundation, and family as she awaited the miracle of a liver transplant and how God got her through it all. She said, "God motivated me to share my story with others who may be going through a difficult life experience—particularly in the area of a life-threatening illness."

She says, "I am here to encourage you with an uplifting word of faith and give hope to those who feel hopeless. I would not be here if God did not have something amazing for me. All I had to do was to step into my blessing by believing and receiving my miracle from God.

"The Lord has blessed me to be a blessing. To smile and inspired someone, this is reason why God kept me here. I dedicate this book to my wonderful parents, Willie Mann, Jr., Ola B. Mann, and stepmother, Ethel Mann; my lovable husband, Calvin, whom I have been married to for eight years (upon this printing); a marvelous daughter, Nicole Mann, and loving grandchildren Jasmine, Juan, and Joshua. To everyone who has been in my life and touched my heart, "I love you all in Jesus' Name."

www.ingramcontent.com/pod-product-compliance
Lightning Source LLC
Chambersburg PA
CBHW071429180526
45170CB00001B/277